T0227614

The Primary FRCA Structured Oral Examination Study Guide 2

Second Edition

Kate McCombe and Lara Wijayasiri

Illustrations by Paul Hatton • Foreword by David Bogod

CRC Press
Taylor & Francis Group
Boca Raton London New York

CRC Press is an imprint of the
Taylor & Francis Group, an **informa** business

CRC Press
Taylor & Francis Group
6000 Broken Sound Parkway NW, Suite 300
Boca Raton, FL 33487-2742

© 2016 by Taylor & Francis Group, LLC
CRC Press is an imprint of Taylor & Francis Group, an Informa business

No claim to original U.S. Government works

International Standard Book Number-13: 978-1-78523-105-6 (Paperback)

Visit the Taylor & Francis Web site at
http://www.taylorandfrancis.com

and the CRC Press Web site at
http://www.crcpress.com

CONTENTS

PART 02

PART 03

FOREWORD

Much has happened since I wrote the Foreword to the first edition of this invaluable guide to the Primary FRCA Structured Oral Examination in 2010. Of the three original authors, two have married (each other) and produced a baby girl. One of these two has had to relinquish the authorship of this new edition, since his promotion to the ranks of Primary Examiner unsurprisingly bars him from writing a book on how to pass the Primary exam. The two remaining authors have both moved up the ranks and been appointed as consultants, one with an interest in obstetrics, ethics and law, and the other specialising in vascular anaesthesia and the difficult airway. The first edition, meanwhile, has rapidly become the best-selling textbook on the Primary SOE. If a soap opera was ever to be based around the publication of a guide to passing post-graduate anaesthetic exams – admittedly an unlikely proposition – the story of McCombe and Wijayasiri would surely rival 'EastEnders' for intrigue and plot development.

In this new edition, as well as updating existing topics, the authors have included substantial additions to what was already a very comprehensive book, in line with changes made by the Royal College to the Primary syllabus. The section on 'special patient groups' now includes paediatrics and the elderly, the latter of increasingly personal interest to this writer. The section on physics – often a stumbling block for the Primary candidate – has been extensively revised and now covers those perennial favourites of the examiners, arterial waveforms and vaporisers; as one reads these, there are frequent 'aha!' moments, not least with respect to critical damping, the pumping effect and the influence of altitude on performance. Mindful of the old adage that 'a picture paints a thousand words', the authors have enhanced the number and quality of diagrams and figures, helping to clarify areas such as fetal circulation and the Kreb's cycle.

Some aspects of these books remain, thankfully, unchanged, in particular the resolutely pragmatic approach that McCombe and Wijayasiri take to help readers through the tangled thickets of the Primary. Here are the questions the examiners like to ask, the authors seem to say, and this is how to answer them. It is, perhaps, a tribute to the exam syllabus itself that this approach results in a textbook that is not only very readable but also highly educational.

In short, if you are not lucky enough to be working in the same hospital as the authors and you cannot approach them for viva practice (or even if you can), then the new edition of this book is an essential companion and a true *vade mecum*. Look it up – a bit of Latin can still impress the examiners!

David Bogod
Consultant Anaesthetist and Ex-Editor-in-Chief of *Anaesthesia*
Nottingham

PREFACE

During our revision for the primary exam we were advised that the best way to ensure success in the structured oral examination (SOE) was to prepare answers to all of the questions in the back of *The Royal College of Anaesthetists Guide to the FRCA Examination, The Primary*. Undoubtedly, this was excellent advice but it proved an enormous task and one we simply did not have time to complete before our own exams. However, once they were over, we began to answer all those questions in the hope that this might help others to prepare for the Primary, or for the basic science component of the Final FRCA. Finally then, here is the result: the book we wish we'd had.

The Primary FRCA Structured Oral Examination Study Guide provides answers to the questions regularly posed by the examiners. We have not attempted to write the next great anaesthetic textbook, but rather to collate information and deliver it in a relevant and userfriendly layout to make your exam preparation a little easier.

In the SOE itself, each topic will be examined for approximately five minutes. Many of these answers contain much more information than could reasonably be expected of you in that time; however, we have tried to cover several angles of questioning.

We have included the usual chapters on physiology, pharmacology (*Study Guide 1*) and physics (*Study Guide 2*) and, in addition, have written a section on patients who present the anaesthetist with unique problems, 'special patient groups' (*Study Guide 2*). These patients tend to appear in the clinical SOE before some terrible 'critical incident' befalls them. Again, we have included a section addressing the 'critical incidents' beloved of the examiner, with advice as to how to approach them in the SOE (*Study Guide 2*).

There is a unique pharmacology section including information on drugs commonly examined presented in a spider diagram layout. These extremely visual learning aids allowed us to revise the drugs in the necessary detail, and helped us to recall the information even under the acute stress of the exam. We hope you find them just as useful.

We wish you every success in what is undoubtedly a rigorous exam. We believe the key to this success is to practise presenting the knowledge that you already have, logically and concisely. The only way to do this is to practise speaking, even though the possibility of exposing any ignorance is daunting. The more you talk, the more you will cover, and every question is so much easier to answer in the exam if you have already had a dress rehearsal. We hope this book will help you in your preparations.

Good luck!

Lara Wijayasiri
Kate McCombe
December 2015

To Andrew, who makes me believe anything is possible.

Kate McCombe

To Amish, my husband and best friend- thank you for giving me the time to complete this book. And to Maya, my beautiful daughter- thank you for giving me a greater focus in life other than this book.

Lara Wijayasiri

CONTRIBUTORS

Paul Hatton B.Tec
Illustrations

Dr Barbara Lattuca MBBCh MRCP FRCA
Locum Consultant Anaesthetist, St George's NHS Healthcare Trust

Pharmacology
> Drugs and the kidney
> Inhalational anaesthetic agents (volatile agents)
> Antiplatelet agents
> Hypoglycaemic agents
> Antidepressants

Special patient groups
> Diabetes

Lt Col Mark Wyldbore MBBS BSc(Hons) FRCA RAMC
Consultant Anaesthetist, Queen Victoria Hospital NHS Foundation Trust

Pharmacology
> Drugs and the liver
> Total intravenous anaesthesia
> Anticoagulants

ACKNOWLEDGEMENT

Dr Tim Case MBBChir MPhil MA(Cantab)
Our sincerest thanks go to Tim for his eagle eyes and enviable grasp of physics. The book is better for his meticulous reading and attention to detail!

Part 01

PHARMACOLOGY

1. RECEPTORS

Define 'receptor' and 'ligand'.		**Receptors** are proteins, usually integral to the cell membrane, with selective ligand-binding sites.
		A **ligand** is any substance able to bind to a receptor and bring about biological change within the cell. A ligand may be capable of binding to more than one receptor and exerting different effects at each different one.
What governs drug–receptor interactions?		The **law of mass action** governs drug–receptor interactions and so the rate of interaction is proportional to the concentration of drug and receptor. It is a specific, dose-dependent and saturatable interaction.

What are the different classes of receptors?

Table 1.1   Receptor classes

Receptor	Ligand-gated ion channel receptor	G-protein-coupled receptor	Tyrosine kinase linked receptor	Intracel- lular nuclear receptors
Location	Membrane	Membrane	Membrane	Cytosol
Effector	Channel	Enzyme/Channel	Tyrosine kinase	Gene transcription
Coupling	Direct	G protein	Direct	via DNA
Speed	Milliseconds	Seconds	Minutes	Hours
Examples	nAChR GABA$_A$	mAChR Adrenoceptors	Insulin receptor	Thyroxine receptor Steroid receptor

What are the main mechanisms of receptor action?

> **Altered ion permeability:**
>   • Acetylcholine (ACh) binds to the two α subunits of the pentameric nicotinic acetylcholine receptor (nAChR), causing a conformational change, which opens a central pore allowing an influx of Na^+ ions, leading to cell depolarisation.

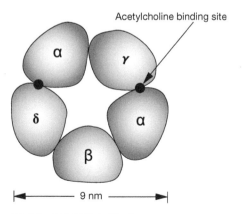

Fig. 1.1   Acetylcholine receptor

- Benzodiazepines bind to a specific site on the $GABA_A$ receptor, causing a conformational change, which opens a central pore allowing an influx of Cl^- ions, leading to cell hyperpolarisation.

> **Intermediate (secondary) messengers:**
  - There are several types of secondary messengers including cyclic adenosine monophosphate (cAMP), cyclic guanosine monophosphate (cGMP), inositol triphosphate (IP_3), diacylglycerol (DAG) and calcium ions (Ca^{2+}).
  - These are involved in signal transduction and signal amplification, and the rate of production of these second messengers is altered by a ligand binding to a G-protein-coupled receptor (GPCR).
  - They have a diverse effect on the cell by activation of protein kinases and modulation of calcium channels.
  - cAMP is activated by G_s proteins (e.g. via stimulation of β adrenoceptors and glucagon receptors).
  - cAMP is inhibited by G_i proteins (e.g. via stimulation of α_2 adrenoceptors and opioid receptors).
  - IP_3 and DAG are activated by G_q proteins (e.g. via stimulation of α_1 adrenoceptors and muscarinic acetylcholine receptors).
  - cGMP is activated by nitric oxide.

> **Regulation of gene transcription:**
  - These receptors are located intracellularly and are targeted by lipid-soluble ligands, typically hormones (e.g. thyroxine and steroids), that can diffuse easily into the cell.
  - Once in the cytosol, the ligands bind with receptors and then the ligand–receptor complex enters the nucleus, alters DNA transcription and therefore protein synthesis.
  - This system operates over a matter of hours, which explains why it takes 6–8 hours to achieve a clinical response following hydrocortisone administration in acute asthma.

What is the structure of the G-protein-coupled receptor (GPCR)?

> GPCR consists of seven α helices, which span the cell membrane forming an extracellular site (where the ligand binds) and an intracellular site (where the G protein attaches).
> Each GPCR can be associated with up to a hundred G proteins, which promotes signal amplification.

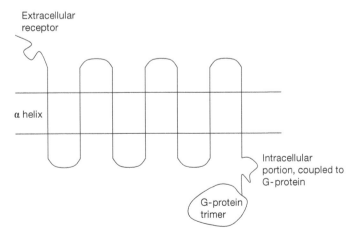

Fig. 1.2 Schematic representation of a G-protein coupled receptor

What are G proteins?

> G proteins (or GTP-binding proteins) are regulatory proteins, which couple the activation of a surface receptor to the activation of an intracellular enzyme (e.g. adenylate cyclase) so that a secondary messenger can be produced (e.g. cAMP), allowing signal transduction and amplification to occur.
> They are heterotrimeric proteins (i.e. they consist of α, β and γ subunits, which join together to form a trimer).

Which different types of G proteins are there?

> The main types of G proteins are the 'stimulatory' (i.e. G_s and G_q) and the 'inhibitory' (i.e. G_i) proteins.
> G_s proteins stimulate adenylate cyclase, causing a rise in cAMP (e.g. β adrenoceptors and glucagon receptor).
> G_q proteins stimulate phospholipase C, causing a rise in IP_3 and DAG (e.g. α_1 adrenoceptor and muscarinic acetylcholine receptor (mAChR)).
> G_i proteins inhibit adenylate cyclase, causing a fall in cAMP (e.g. α_2 adrenoceptors and opioid receptors).

What happens when a GPCR is activated?

> When a ligand binds to the extracellular site of a GPCR, it causes a GTP molecule to bind to the intracellular α subunit of the G-protein trimer.
> This causes a conformational change within the trimer, resulting in its separation from the receptor and dissociation into a $\beta\gamma$ and an α-GTP complex.
> The α-GTP complex then goes on to activate (or inhibit) the various enzymes systems (e.g. adenylate cyclase, guanylate cyclase and phospholipase C) resulting in the production of the secondary messengers.
> The α subunit has intrinsic GTPase activity and so it converts the GTP into GDP.
> Once the α subunit is bound only to GDP, it rejoins the $\beta\gamma$ units to return to its resting state. The reformed G-protein trimer reattaches to the intracellular portion of the receptor and the receptor system is ready to be stimulated once again.

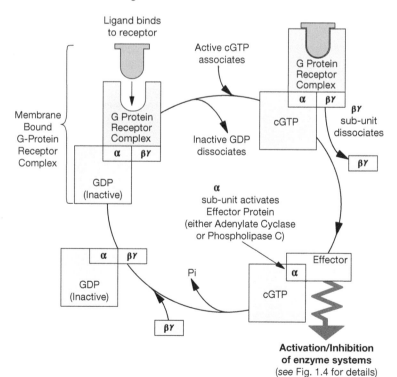

Fig. 1.3 Activation of G-protein coupled receptor

Fig. 1.4   Effects of activating G-protein coupled receptor

2. MECHANISM OF DRUG ACTION

How do drugs work?

Drugs produce their effects by acting on numerous different systems within the body. Below is a list of the effecter sites at which drugs act, along with some clinical examples.

Receptors
> Ligand-gated ion channels
  * Suxamethonium is an agonist at nAChR while rocuronium is an antagonist.
  * Diazepam is an agonist at $GABA_A$ receptors while flumazenil is an antagonist.
> G-protein-coupled receptors
  * Dobutamine is an agonist at β-adrenoceptors while atenolol is an antagonist.
  * Morphine is an agonist at opioid receptors while naloxone is an antagonist.
> Tyrosine kinase receptors
  * Insulin is an agonist at insulin receptors.
> Intracellular receptors
  * Hydrocortisone is an agonist at steroid receptors.

Ion channels
  * Lignocaine blocks the fast Na^+ channels.
  * Verapamil blocks L-type Ca^{2+} channels.

Enzymes
  * Neostigmine inhibits acetylcholinesterase.
  * Aspirin inhibits cyclo-oxygenase 1 and 2.

Hormones
  * Carbimazole reduces thyroxine production.
  * Metformin increases insulin production.

Neurotransmitters
  * Ephedrine increases presynaptic noradrenaline release.
  * Amitriptyline and cocaine reduce noradrenaline reuptake.

Transport systems
  * Digoxin inhibits the cardiac Na^+/K^+ ATPase pump.
  * Furosemide inhibits the $Na^+/K^+/2Cl^-$ ATPase pump in the loop of Henle.

Physicochemical
  * Sugammadex chelates rocuronium.
  * Antacids neutralise gastric acids.

3. DRUG INTERACTIONS

What is a drug interaction?	> A drug interaction occurs when the action of one drug is altered by the concurrent or prior administration of another drug. > It is estimated that one in six drug charts contains a significant drug interactions. This is becoming increasingly significant as many patients are on multiple drugs, some of which can interfere with anaesthetic agents.
How can drug interactions be classified?	> **Physicochemical** drug interactions occur due to the physical properties of the drugs themselves. > **Pharmacokinetic** drug interactions occur when one drug alters the way in which the body handles another. > **Pharmacodynamic** drug interactions occur when the action of one drug is altered by the administration of another.

Give examples of physicochemical drug interactions you may encounter.	Some drug interactions are clinically useful:
	> **Chelation**
	  • Sugammadex and rocuronium
	> **Neutralisation**
	  • Heparin and protamine
	
	Others occur inadvertently with undesirable effects:
	> **Precipitation**
	  • Thiopentone (weak acid) and suxamethonium (weak base)
	> **Adsorption**
	  • Halothane dissolving into rubber

Give examples of pharmacokinetic drug interactions.	These drug interactions can affect drug absorption, distribution, metabolism and excretion.
	
	> Absorption
	  • Adrenaline administered with local anaesthetics reduces absorption of the local anaesthetic by causing local vasoconstriction
	> Distribution
	  • Aspirin (80% plasma protein bound) displaces warfarin (97% plasma protein bound) from plasma proteins, thereby increasing the unbound fraction of warfarin and increasing the risk of bleeding.
	> Metabolism
	  • Phenytoin, carbamazepine, rifampicin and barbiturates induce hepatic enzymes, which results in the accelerated breakdown of drugs metabolised by these enzymes.
	  • Omeprazole and cimetidine inhibit hepatic enzymes, reducing the breakdown of drugs metabolised by these enzymes.
	> Excretion
	  • Alkalinising the urine increases the renal excretion of salicylates.

Give examples of pharmacodynamic drug interactions.

> **Summation** occurs when the action of two or more drugs is additive (i.e. 1 + 1 = 2):
> • nitrous oxide and inhalational anaesthetic agents.
> **Synergism** occurs when the combined action of two or more drugs is greater than the sum of their individual effects (i.e. 1 + 1 > 2):
> • propofol and remifentanil
> **Potentiation** occurs when the action of one drug is increased by the administration of another drug:
> • probenecid increases the action of penicillin by reducing its renal excretion
> **Antagonism** occurs when the action of one drug is blocked or reversed by another drug (i.e. 1 + 1 = 0):
> • morphine and naloxone.

4. DRUG ABSORPTION AND BIOAVAILABILITY

What factors influence drug absorption?

Drug absorption describes the passage of a drug into the bloodstream from its route of administration. Factors influencing this are as follows:

> **Route of administration**
> **Particle size**
> **pK$_a$ and ionisation:** Unionised drugs cross membranes more readily (*see* below).
> **Lipid solubility:** The more lipid soluble a drug, the more readily it can cross the phospholipid bilayer of cells, and the faster it is absorbed.
> **Concentration gradient:** The higher the concentration gradient between the lumen containing the 'drug load' and the cells into which it is diffusing, the faster it will be absorbed.
> **Other factors:** Bacterial overgrowth will reduce drug absorption and some drugs will be affected by intake of other substances, e.g. milk chelates tetracycline antibiotics and so decreases their availability for absorption.

How can manufacturers alter rate of drug absorption?

Most drugs are taken orally and pass from the mouth into the aqueous and acidic environment of the stomach. Here they may dissolve and cross into the cells lining the stomach. Dissolution and absorption can be altered by the manufacturers in several ways:

> **Particle size:** The larger the particle size (molecular weight) of the drug, the more slowly it will dissolve.
> **Compounds used:** Different compounds dissolve at different rates. Modified-release or slow-release drugs can improve the drug profile, minimising peaks and troughs in plasma concentration. Patient compliance improves with less frequent dosing.
> **Coating the tablet:** Enteric coating does not dissolve in acid conditions and therefore the drug will pass to the basic intestine before dissolving.

What are the available routes for drug administration?

> Enteral (variable availability: formulation of drug, pK$_a$, gastric pH, GI transit time, etc.)
> Intravenous (bioavailability is taken as 1.0 or 100%)
> Transdermal (suitable for small, potent, lipophilic drugs)
> Intranasal (rich blood supply, avoids first-pass metabolism, variable absorption: mucus flow etc.)
> Sublingual (rich blood supply, avoids first-pass metabolism, variable absorption: saliva flow, swallowing etc.)
> Intrapulmonary (conduit for volatile agents to lungs: large surface area, rich blood supply)
> Intramuscular (variable absorption: regional blood flow, injections can be formulated for slow release)

> Epidural (reduced systemic absorption in general, localised effect though beware, opioids may still cause respiratory depression)
> Subarachnoid (as above)
> Rectal (avoids first-pass metabolism, useful when nausea and vomiting problematic)
> Vaginal (avoids first-pass metabolism, limited systemic absorption, primarily used to administer drugs whose action is on vagina/nearby structures)

What is pK_a and how does this influence drug absorption?

Before answering this question, a reminder of some basic concepts:

> An **acid** is a proton (H^+ ion) donor.
> A **base** is a proton acceptor (OH^-).
> A **weak acid/base** is one that dissociates in water to form an equilibrium with its ions, e.g. $H_2CO_3 \rightleftharpoons H^+ \rightleftharpoons HCO_3^-$.
> A **strong acid/base** is one that dissociates very readily and does not form an equilibrium, e.g. $HCl \rightarrow H^+ + Cl^-$.
> An amphoteric compound has the ability to behave as an acid or a base, e.g. water (in some senses, all compounds are amphoteric as they can always be (de)protonated by a stronger acid/base).
> The K_a is the dissociation constant and it describes how readily an acid in solution gives up its hydrogen ions.
> It describes the ratio of the products of the reaction, to the concentration of the initial reactants.
> It is written:

$$K_a = \frac{[A^-][H^+]}{[HA]}$$

where HA is the acid, A^- is its conjugate base (i.e. the product that is now able to accept protons) and H^+ its proton. The higher the value of K_a, the more readily the acid gives up its proton and dissociates.

> K_a can be expressed in its logarithmic form giving us the pK_a.
> pK_a is the negative log of the acid dissociation constant, and is defined as $-\log_{10} K_a$.
> pK_a is used because it yields more convenient units that are easier to use for practical purposes.
> The pK_a of a drug is the pH at which it is exactly half dissociated, i.e. the drug is 50% ionised and 50% unionised.
> The larger the value of pK_a, the less readily the acid dissociates to donate its H^+ ion at a given pH, i.e. the weaker the acid. Conversely, the smaller the value of pK_a, the more readily the acid donates its proton and the stronger the acid.

> *Most drugs are either weak acids or weak bases. Unfortunately, you cannot tell from the pK$_a$ of a drug whether it is basic or acidic; this is a property of each drug you just have to learn.*

	Bases	pK$_a$	Acids	pK$_a$	
Weak	Diazepam	3.7	Salicylic Acid	3	Strong
	Etomidate	4.1	Frusemide	3.9	
	Midazolam	6.15			
	Alfentanil	6.5			
	Ketamine	7.5	Thiopentone	7.6	
	Lignocaine	7.8	Methohexitone	7.9	
	Bupivacaine	8.2	Atropine	8.9	
	Fentanyl	8.4	Paracetamol	9.5	
	Morphine	8.6			
Strong			Propofol	11	Weak

Fig. 4.1 pK$_a$ values of some basic and acidic drugs

At pH < pK$_a$, acidic drugs become less ionised:

$$HA \rightleftharpoons H^+ + A^-$$

Putting the acidic drug in a more acidic environment raises H^+ concentration and so drives the equation to the left.

At pH < pK$_a$, basic drugs become more ionised as they accept protons:

$$B + H^+ \rightleftharpoons BH^+$$

Putting a basic drug in an acidic environment drives the equation to the right as the base (B) 'accepts' the protons.

Drugs cross membranes in the un-ionised state and so their pK$_a$ and the pH of the surrounding environment affect their rate of absorption. Hence, acidic drugs will be more readily absorbed in the highly acidic stomach, whereas basic drugs are better absorbed in the intestine where pH is higher.

Relationship between pH and the percentage of drug in the un-ionised form, for (a) a weak acid (thiopentone: pK_a 7.6) and (b) a weak base (fentanyl: pK_a 8.4)

Fig. 4.2 pH vs. degree of ionisation for thiopentone and fentanyl

What is the Henderson–Hasselbalch equation and how is it useful in predicting drug absorption?

> The Henderson–Hasselbalch equation describes the derivation of pH as a measure of acidity. pH is calculated using the pK_a and the equation can be expressed in two ways:

$$pH = pK_a + \log\frac{[\text{conjugate base}]}{[\text{acid}]}$$

$$pH = pK_a + \log\frac{[A^-]}{[HA]}$$

Where pK_a is $-\log(K_a)$.

> Using the non-specific acid–base reaction: $HA + H_2O \rightleftharpoons A^- + H_3O^+$ pK_a can be substituted into the equation, to give the Henderson–Hasselbalch equation:

$$-\log(K_a) = -\log\frac{[H_3O^+][A^-]}{HA}$$

> This is used to calculate:
  • pH of a solution
  • pH at which the equation is in equilibrium and the drug exists as 50% ionised and unionised, i.e. the pK_a of the drug, proportions of ionised and un-ionised drug in a solution at a given pH.

Define bioavailability.

> Bioavailability describes the fraction of the drug administered that reaches the bloodstream.
> If a drug is given intravenously it is introduced straight into the bloodstream and is said to have a bioavailability of 1 or 100%.
> For drugs given orally, the bioavailability is calculated by comparing the plasma concentration of the drug when administered orally to the plasma concentration when it is administered intravenously. This is achieved by comparing the area under the curve (AUC) of the two conditions:

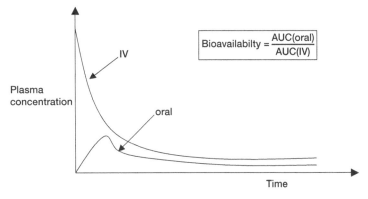

$$\text{Bioavailabilty} = \frac{AUC(oral)}{AUC(IV)}$$

Fig. 4.3 Plasma concentrations of a drug administered intravenously and orally

What is first-pass metabolism?

> This refers to the process by which drugs absorbed from the gastrointestinal tract enter the hepatic portal circulation and are carried to the liver. The liver then metabolises the drug such that only a fraction of the original dose is returned to the systemic circulation.
> Drugs that undergo extensive first-pass metabolism have low oral bioavailability and it may be necessary to find an alternative route of administration that allows the drug to enter the systemic circulation directly.

Can you give examples of drugs that undergo first-pass metabolism?

> Aspirin (70%)
> Codeine (60%)
> Morphine (40%)
> Diltiazem (40%)
> Propranolol (30%)
> Verapamil (20%)
> Hydralazine (15–30%)

5. DRUGS AND THE LIVER

In which ways are drugs metabolised by the liver?

The metabolism of drugs in the liver is defined as the modification or degradation of drugs in order to activate, deactivate, toxify or detoxify drugs in the body.

The majority of metabolic reactions serve to de-activate and aid the excretion of the drugs, often by turning a lipophilic compound to a readily excreted polar one (*see* Chapter 6: 'Drugs and the kidney').

The rate at which the drug is metabolised will be an important factor in the intensity and duration of the drug's action.

Some drugs are given as pro-drugs that need to be metabolised in order to become active, e.g. enalapril, which must be converted to enalaprilat for its action. Others may have active substrates, such as morphine, or substrates with completely different actions.

How are drugs metabolised by the liver?

The types of reaction that occur can be classified into phase I or phase II reactions. While they may occur in other parts of the body, the majority take place in the smooth endoplasmic reticulum of liver.

Phase I reactions:
> These normally precede phase II reactions and involve oxidation, reduction or hydrolysis of the drug in order to activate or deactivate it.
> The reaction usually adds or unmasks polar bodies in the chemical.
> Oxidation and reduction are mainly hepatic, whereas hydrolysis is more widespread throughout the body, e.g. by plasma cholinesterase.
> For oxidation reactions the cytochrome P450 system of enzymes is particularly important. These enzymes show genetic variability and their activity can be induced or inhibited by the presence of certain other drugs or chemicals (*see* Table 5.1). This becomes of particular importance when the drugs concerned have a narrow therapeutic window and inhibition of their metabolism will cause toxicity, or induction of their metabolism will render them ineffective.
> Drugs undergoing phase 1 reactions include phenothiazines, paracetamol and steroids.
> For some drugs, this reaction will be sufficient to allow excretion, but others will require further modification and undergo phase II reactions.

Table 5.1   List of common drugs that induce or inhibit the hepatic cytochrome P450 enzyme system

Inhibitors	Inducers
Metronidazole	Carbamazepine
Ciprofloxacin	Rifampicin
Fluconazole	Alcohol (Acute intake)
Erythromycin	Phenytoin
Ethanol (Chronic use)	Griseofulvin
Dextroproxyphene (co-proxamol)	Primidone
Cimetidine	Inhalational agents (enflurane, halothane)
Amiodarone	Smoking
Ketoconazole	Barbiturates
Etomidate	Glucocorticoids
Grapefruit	

Phase II reactions:

> These involve adding groups to the drugs and are sometimes referred to as conjugation or synthetic reactions. These groups increase the water solubility of the drugs and allow excretion in the bile or urine. Although they often follow Phase I reactions they may be the only step in the metabolism of drugs.
> Phase II reactions include glucuronidation, sulphation, acetylation and methylation.

Which drugs can cause damage to the liver?

Drug-induced hepatitis can follow acute or chronic drug exposure. The most commonly encountered drug causing direct hepatocellular damage is ethanol. Chronic alcohol abuse in genetically susceptible individuals can cause progressive inflammatory liver damage, which may result in fatty liver and cirrhosis.

Alcohol damages the liver in several ways:

> Ethanol and its metabolite acetaldehyde damage the liver cell and mitochondrial membranes.
> Free radicals, superoxides and hydroperoxides generated during ethanol metabolism damage the liver.
> Alcoholic hepatitis stimulates the immune system, which generates autoantibodies.

The volatile anaesthetic agent halothane is also known to cause hepatitis, with a mortality rate of 50% in those affected.

> Halothane can cause a reversible transaminitis as a result of hepatic hypoxia.
> It can cause significant centrilobular liver necrosis in what appears to be an immune-mediated process.
> Halothane is oxidised, producing trifluroacetyl metabolites, which bind to liver proteins. In genetically susceptible individuals this causes an autoimmune response and antibodies are generated against the complex.
> Risk factors include repeated exposure, female sex, obesity and middle age.

The volatile agents enflurane and isoflurane are also metabolised to acetylated metabolites, but this only involves 2 and 0.2% of the total dose respectively, compared to 20% of halothane.

How does chronic liver disease affect the drugs used in anaesthesia?

> Porto-caval shunts occurring in cirrhosis reduce hepatic blood flow and hence the extraction ratio of the drug. This results in an increased drug bioavailability.
> Impaired production of albumin results in reduced drug plasma protein binding. This leads to an increase in the free, active component of the drug.
> Ascites and the overall increase in total body water leads to an increase in the volume of distribution of drugs.
> Reduced metabolic function (phase I and II reactions) leads to prolonged action of hepatically metabolised drugs.
> Impaired coagulation (the liver synthesises many of the clotting factors) and liver-induced thrombocytopenia may contraindicate the use of central neuroaxial blocks.

Benzodiazepines:	Metabolism impaired and effects enhanced. These drugs should be avoided.
Opiates:	Metabolism impaired and effects enhanced. Use with caution in reduced doses.
Barbiturates:	Metabolism impaired, though their effects are terminated by redistribution.
Suxamethonium:	Duration of action prolonged as decreased plasma cholinesterases.
Muscle relaxants:	Effects enhanced as usually highly protein bound.
	Hoffmann degradation of atracurium may be reduced in the lower pH associated with severe disease.
Fluid:	Extreme care should be used in administering intravenous fluids as oedema and fluid overload are likely. Also avoid lactate-containing fluids, e.g. Hartmann's as lactate metabolism will be impaired.

6. DRUGS AND THE KIDNEY

How are drugs excreted from the body?

> Most drugs are excreted from the body by a combination of metabolism by the liver and excretion via the kidneys.
> Most parent drug molecules and their phase I metabolites are extensively reabsorbed at the level of the kidney tubules, whereas their more water-soluble phase II conjugates are only minimally reabsorbed and readily excreted.
> Some parent drugs are almost exclusively excreted by the kidneys without prior detoxification, such that any alteration in kidney function can result in toxicity. Examples include:
>   • Oxybarbiturates
>   • Gentamicin
>   • Furosemide
>   • Ampicillin
>   • Sotalol
>   • Methotrexate.

Describe how drugs are handled as they pass through the kidney, illustrating your answer with examples.

The kidney affects drug elimination at three main stages:
> Glomerular filtration
> Active proximal tubular secretion
> Passive distal tubular reabsorption

Glomerular filtration
> The rate of filtration is governed by the glomerular filtration rate.
> Drugs that are of low molecular weight (<60 000 Daltons) and that are not plasma protein bound (PPB) are readily filtered, e.g. fluconazole and ofloxacin.
> Most intravenous anaesthetic agents are of low molecular weight but are highly protein bound, e.g. propofol (98% PPB).
> Heparin is a large molecule that cannot be filtered.

Active proximal tubular secretion
> The rate of tubular secretion is governed by renal blood flow.
> It is an energy-dependent process and is carrier mediated.
> Two types of carrier exist:
>   • Those for acidic drugs, e.g. furosemide, penicillin, nonsteroidal anti-inflammatory drugs (NSAIDs) and glucuronide and sulphate conjugates
>   • Those for basic drugs, e.g. histamine and dopamine
> Tubular secretion is more important for acidic rather than basic drugs.
> Many drugs are actively secreted from the renal blood vessels into the proximal tubules because most of the renal blood flow (80%) escapes filtration by the glomeruli, e.g. angiotensin-converting enzyme (ACE) inhibitors and penicillin.
> Some drugs compete for the same carriers and limit the other's secretion, e.g. probenecid administered with penicillin and sulphonamides administered with indomethacin.
> Tubular secretion can secrete drugs against their concentration gradients. It is an efficient system even for highly protein-bound drugs.

Passive distal tubular reabsorption

> As water is reabsorbed along the tubule, the drug's increasing concentration gradient drives the process of passive reabsorption.
> Highly lipid-soluble drugs, e.g. fentanyl, are reabsorbed into the circulation as they pass down the distal convoluted tubule.
> Some drugs are too lipid insoluble to undergo reabsorption, e.g. digoxin, aminoglycoside antibiotics, and glucuronide and sulphate conjugates from phase II metabolism.
> Changes in urine pH can alter the tubular reabsorption of weakly acidic or basic drugs by altering their degree of ionisation and consequently their lipid solubility. This, in turn, affects their speed of elimination.
> Weak bases become more ionised (lipid insoluble) in acidic urine and therefore less well reabsorbed.
> Weak acids become more ionised in alkaline urine. This is applied clinically in the administration of sodium bicarbonate to alkalinise the urine in overdoses of aspirin and phenobarbital.

What are the effects of age on renal drug metabolism?

Renal function, notably GFR decreases with age.

> Increasing age is associated with progressive loss of kidney structure and function with decreases in glomerular filtration rate (GFR) and renal blood flow (RBF).
> Consequently, drug elimination is reduced, and the elderly are at increased risk of acute renal failure in the post-operative period.
> GFR (140 ml/min/1.73 m^2 in adulthood) and thus creatinine clearance declines by about 8 ml/min/1.73 m^2 per decade after the age of 40.
> Serum creatinine remains within the normal range because although less is excreted, less creatinine is also produced (less muscle mass and less physical activity).
> RBF is well maintained at 500–600 ml/min until the fourth decade, and then declines by about 10% per decade.

Both structural and haemodynamic changes are responsible.

> Haemodynamic changes:
>   • Reduced glomerular capillary plasma flow rate
>   • Reduced glomerular capillary ultrafiltration coefficient (due to reductions in both the glomerular capillary permeability and the surface area available for filtration)
>   • Reduction in afferent arteriolar resistance, with an increase in glomerular capillary hydraulic pressure, and accompanying proteinuria and progressive glomerular sclerosis.

> Structural changes:
>   • Reduced renal mass, in particular the cortex (adult kidney 400 g, declines by eighth decade to 300 g)
>   • Reduced number of glomeruli (absolute and functional)
>   • Hyalinisation of afferent arterioles
>   • Development of aglomerular arterioles (direct channels between the afferent and efferent arterioles)
>   • Increased percentage of sclerotic glomeruli (5% by 30 years; 30% by 80 years)
>   • Tubulointerstitial fibrosis.

In addition, ageing is associated with other systemic changes that contribute to reductions in RBF and GFR:

> Altered cardiovascular haemodynamics (reduced cardiac output and increased systemic blood pressure)
> Altered responsiveness to vasoactive stimuli (vasoconstrictor responses are enhanced, while vasodilatory responses are impaired).

Examples of drugs where elimination may be significantly affected

The above changes decrease renal elimination of many drugs and doses or their frequency needs adjusting:

> Analgesics: morphine, remifentanil, oxycodone, gabapentin
> Neuromuscular blocking agents: aminosteroid group (vecuronium > rocuronium > pancuronium)
> Neuromuscular blocking agent antagonists: neostigmine and sugammadex
> Cardiovascular drugs: ACE inhibitors, digoxin
> Diuretics: furosemide, thiazides, amiloride
> Antibiotics: amikacin, gentamicin, ciprofloxacin, levofloxacin, streptomycin.

Most other anaesthetic agents and adjuvant drugs require dose adjustments in the elderly for reasons other than reduced renal elimination.

7. VARIATIONS IN DRUG METABOLISM

What factors can cause a variable biological response to drugs amongst patients?

There are several factors that affect drug handling in different patient groups, for example:

> Age, e.g. elderly patients are often volume deplete and so volume of distribution of drug may be decreased.
> Race, e.g. there is evidence that ACE inhibitors are less effective at treating heart failure in black patients than in white.
> Sex, e.g. men have higher levels of alcohol dehydrogenase than women
> Disease state, e.g. in liver disease decreased production of plasma. proteins may alter drug binding; cancer, obesity, heart failure and infection among other things can alter the activity of drug-metabolising enzymes.
> Genetic polymorphism – *see* below.

Explain how genetic polymorphism influences drug metabolism. What clinical effects can this have?

This question is a clear lead into a discussion about suxamethonium apnoea, but do not forget about other drugs whose actions are also affected by the recipient's genetics.

Genetic polymorphism is a term that describes the difference in people's genotype and subsequent variation in phenotypic expression of these genes. The enzymes that metabolise drugs are subject to genetic polymorphism, and so there can be differences between individuals in the handling of the same drug.

> **Suxamethonium:**
> • Suxamethonium is broken down by plasma cholinesterases.
> • These enzymes are coded for by autosomal genes on chromosome 3. The normal phenotype is Eu (usual). A patient with Eu:Eu will break down suxamethonium rapidly so that its duration of action is around 2–6 minutes.
> • There are several variations of these genes and deviation from the normal means that the resulting enzyme's activity is decreased. Consequently, it takes longer to break down the suxamethonium and its duration of action is increased.
> • Abnormal forms of the gene include Ea (atypical), Es (silent) and Ef (fluoride resistant).
> • The most common abnormality is Ea:Eu. This is carried by 4% of the Caucasian population, and their recovery time following suxamethonium is extended to around 30 minutes. The incidence of this phenotype is higher in Asians and lower in Afro-Caribbeans.

Incidence and prolongation of block:

Ea:Ea	1/3000	≥2 hours
Ef: Ef	1/100 000	≥3 hours
Es:Es	1/250 000	≥3 hours

How would you manage someone with unexpected suxamethonium apnoea?

> The problem should be recognised by the lack of muscle contractions in response to supramaximal nerve stimulation applied several minutes after giving an intubating dose of suxamethonium.
> If the problem has gone unrecognised during surgery and anaesthesia is turned off at the end of the case, the patient's heart rate and BP might rise as an indicator of awareness in the face of sustained paralysis.
> The patient should remain anaesthetised and ventilated until they are able to take good tidal volumes independently.
> FFP could be given theoretically to provide normal plasma cholinesterase. However, the risks of giving it cannot be justified in this situation, instead the patient should remain anaesthetised until the effects of suxamethonium have 'worn off'.
> The patient and their family should be referred for genetic testing to ascertain their phenotype and the extent of any abnormality.

How is the enzyme abnormality diagnosed?

The diagnosis and extent of the enzyme abnormality can be made using dibucaine.

> Dibucaine is a local anaesthetic agent that inhibits normal plasma cholinesterase by approximately 80%, but does not inhibit an abnormal enzyme as effectively.
> Benzylcholine is a substrate broken down by plasma cholinesterase.
> Benzylcholine is added to the plasma sample being tested and the degree of benzylcholine breakdown is measured. If the plasma of a normal patient has benzylcholine solution added to it, it emits a certain wavelength of light, which can be measured. If dibucaine is added to this solution the reaction is inhibited and so less light is emitted. In patients with an abnormal enzyme, dibucaine does not inhibit the reaction as much and so light continues to be emitted.
> The dibucaine number is the percentage inhibition of benzylcholine breakdown by plasma cholinesterase in the presence of dibucaine. A normal number is between 75 and 85, whereas abnormal homozygotes can have numbers as low as 30.

Which other esterases are relevant to anaesthetic practice?

> Plasma esterases rapidly metabolise esmolol. This non-saturatable enzyme system is responsible for esmolol's short duration of action.
> Tissue and plasma esterases rapidly metabolise remifentanil. Again, this non-saturatable enzyme system ensures the rapid breakdown of remifentanil and its context-insensitive half-life.
> Red blood cell esterases metabolise aspirin and diamorphine

What other drugs are affected by genetic polymorphism?

> Mivacurium is also metabolised by plasma cholinesterases and so is subject to the same variations in metabolism as suxamethonium.
> The metabolism of codeine to morphine depends on the enzymes CYZ2D6 and 2C19. There are three broad groups of codeine metabolism:
>   • Poor metabolisers – get little symptomatic relief from codeine (1–7% of the Caucasian population)
>   • Extensive metabolisers – get good relief
>   • Ultra-extensive metabolisers – get very good relief and may be at risk of opioid toxicity (1–7% of the Caucasian population).
> Alcohol is broken down by alcohol dehydrogenase. The expression of this enzyme varies between sexes and races. Men express more than women and therefore can metabolise alcohol more rapidly. European races express an allele that makes their enzyme more active than that of Asians.

8. ISOMERS

What are isomers?	Isomers are molecules that have the same molecular formula but whose atoms are arranged differently. The word comes from the Greek words 'isos' meaning 'equal', and 'meros' meaning 'part'.
How can isomers be classified?	Isomers can be classified as follows:

Fig. 8.1 Classification of isomers

What are structural isomers?

These are compounds that have the same molecular formula but different chemical structures (i.e. their atoms are arranged differently). There are four main forms of structural isomers:

> Chain isomers – carbon skeleton varies but the functional group remains in the same position
> Positional isomers – carbon skeleton remains the same but the functional group varies position
> Functional – carbon skeleton remains the same but the functional group changes
> Tautomers – *see* below.

Isomers may or may not have similar properties depending on the arrangement of their functional groups, e.g. enflurane and isoflurane.

Fig. 8.2 isomers enflurane and isoflurane

What is tautomerism?

This is a form of dynamic isomerism where two structural isomers (known as tautomers) exist in equilibrium. The position of the equilibrium between the two forms depends on the conditions of the surrounding environment.

> Midazolam, which has a seven-membered ring:
>   • pH <4.0 – ring open and water soluble
>   • pH >4.0 – ring closed and lipid soluble.
> Thiopentone isomers alternate between ketone and enol states.
> Morphine isomers alternate between ketone and enol states.

What are stereoisomers?

These are compounds that have the same molecular formula and chemical structure but different spatial arrangements. There are two main forms of stereoisomers:

- enantiomers and diastereoisomers (optical isomers)
- *cis–trans* isomers (geometric isomers).

Enantiomers (previously called 'optical isomers'):

- They possess a single chiral centre (usually carbon or nitrogen atom) to which four other atoms are bonded.
- They form the mirror image of each other but cannot be superimposed upon each other.
- They have identical physical and chemical properties.
- They rotate polarised light equally but in opposite directions (they used to be classified as laevo– or dextro– depending on which way they rotated light).
- Each enantiomer is either the R (rectus) or S (sinister) form. This reflects the direction of ascending atomic number of the atoms attached to the chiral centre. (Imagine sticking the 'limb' with the lowest atomic number into the page. Looking down at the molecule, you would now see three groups sticking up. Count from their highest to the lowest atomic number. If the numbers descend in a clockwise direction, the isomer is the R form, if anti-clockwise, it is an S isomer).
- Examples include levobupivacaine and S-bupivacaine, zopiclone and eszopiclone, citalopram and escitalopram, and ketamine and S-ketamine.

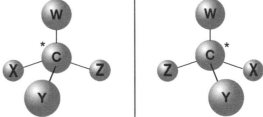

* = chiral centre

Fig. 8.3 Enantiomers

Interestingly, thalidomide is an enantiomer; one form gives the desired antiemetic effect, but the other is responsible for the teratogenic side effects. While the drug companies in the 1970s realised this, they did not appreciate that a proportion of the safe enantiomer is converted to the toxic form in vivo, and so marketed it with catastrophic effect. Thalidomide is being used again as a chemotherapy agent.

Diastereoisomers:
- They possess more than one chiral centre and so they cannot form mirror images of each other.
- Examples include atracurium, which has four chiral centres.

***Cis–trans* isomers** (previously called 'geometric isomers'):
- They possess a double bond around which the attached atoms cannot rotate.
- *Cis*-form – the groups are arranged on the same side of the double bond.
- *Trans*-form – the groups are arranged on opposite sides of the double bond.

- An example is mivacurium where 36% is *cis–trans*, 58% *trans–trans* and 6% *cis–cis*.
- The *cis–trans* nomenclature only works if the two groups around the double bond are identical.

H₃C   CH₃
   \   /
    C = C
   /   \
  H   H

cis – 2 – butene

H   CH₃
 \   /
  C = C
 /   \
H₃C   H

trans – 2 – butene

Fig. 8.4   *Cis–trans* isomerism

This is a basic review of isomerism, which is sufficient for the exam. There are many other forms of isomerism, which are not discussed and, as far as we know, have not been examined. For example, there are spin isomers whose constituent atoms exhibit different spin characteristics and topoisomers, large molecules that may fold and coil in different ways, e.g. DNA.

What is the clinical relevance of isomerism?

Isomers may have the same molecular formulae and physical properties (e.g. melting points, pK_a, solubility, etc.), butthe altered arrangement of atoms confers different pharmacodynamic/kinetic properties. Some examples are given below:

- Comparing S-ketamine (also called esketamine) with racemic ketamine, S-ketamine has greater affinity for the NMDA receptor, it is twice as potent, patients report a more pleasant experience at doses causing the same effect and recovery of mental function is quicker.
- Comparing esomeprazole with omeprazole, it has higher bioavailability.
- Comparing S-warfarin with R-warfarin, it is more highly protein bound, its volume of distribution is lower, it is more potent and its half-life is only 32 hours compared to 54 hours for R-warfarin.
- Halothane, enflurane and isoflurane are chiral isomers with differing anaesthetic potency.
- Sotolol is formulated as a racemic mixture but only the L-isomer has any beta-blocking activity.
- Some isomers are unsafe for clinical use, e.g. R-thalidomide is sedative while S-thalidomide is teratogenic; L-dopa is used to treat Parkinson's disease, while D-dopa is not because it causes neutropenia.

9. DRUGS TO DRAW

It is not uncommon for you to be asked to draw out the structure of commonly used anaesthetic drugs. You should be able to draw all of the structures shown here.

2,6 Diisopropylphenol

Fig. 9.1 Propofol

	R_1	R_2	R_3
Long acting (Phenobarbitone)	O	$-CH_2-CH_3$	
Intermediate acting (Pentobarbitone)	O	$-CH_2-CH_3$	$-CH\ CH_2CH_2CH_3$ $\quad\ \ \vert$ $\quad\ \ CH_3$
Short acting (Thiopentone)	S	$-CH_2-CH_3$	$-CH\ CH_2CH_2CH_3$ $\quad\ \ \vert$ $\quad\ \ CH_3$

Fig. 9.2 Barbiturates

Fig. 9.3 Inhalational anaesthetic agents

Isoflurane   Enflurane   Sevoflurane   Desflurane

Fig. 9.4 Acetylcholine

Fig. 9.5 Suxamethonium

Fig. 9.6 Adrenaline

Fig. 9.7 Noradrenaline

Fig. 9.8 Dopamine

Fig. 9.9 Sodium nitroprusside

10. EXPONENTIAL FUNCTIONS

Draw a graph showing how the concentration of an intravenously administered drug varies over time.

The plasma concentration of an intravenously administered drug decreases exponentially over time, giving a negative exponential decay curve.

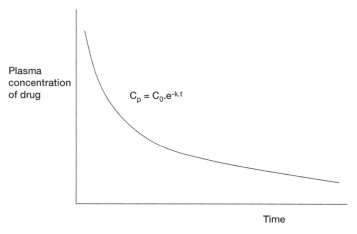

Plasma concentration of drug

$$C_p = C_0.e^{-k.t}$$

Time

Fig. 10.1 Negative exponential decay curve of plasma drug concentration over time

What is an exponential function?

An exponential function describes the situation where the rate of change of quantity of a substance is directly proportional to the quantity of substance at that time. For the graph above this can be equated to:

$$C = dC/dt$$

Where:
C drug concentration
dC change in drug concentration
dt change in time

The formal equation for this negative exponential curve is:

$$C_p = C_0.e^{-k.t}$$

Where:
C_p plasma concentration
C_0 plasma concentration at time zero
e base of natural log
k rate constant
t time

What is 'e'?

e is a mathematical constant and is the base of the natural logarithm. It is sometimes called Euler's number after the Swiss mathematician. Numerically, its value is approximately 2.71828.

What are the properties of an exponential decay curve?

> The plasma concentration approaches, but never touches, the x-axis (i.e. it never becomes zero). Instead, it continues to get closer to the x-axis and reaches a steady state known as an asymptote (this takes approximately five half-lives or three time constants – *see* Chapter 13, 'Volume of distribution, clearance and half-life').
> The absolute amount of drug that is eliminated per minute varies, but the proportion of drug eliminated per minute is constant, e.g. 50% per hour.
> The rate of decline in plasma drug concentration varies according to the plasma concentration of drug present at that time.
> The gradient of the curve is the elimination rate constant, k.

Give some examples of exponential processes.

> **Exponential decay curves:**
>   • Nitrogen washout during pre-oxygenation
>   • Lung volumes during passive expiration
>   • Drug wash-out curves
>   • Radionuclide materials undergoing radioactive decay.
> **Exponential growth curves:**
>   • Bacterial growth
>   • Drug wash-in curves
>   • Lung volumes during positive pressure ventilation (with pressure-controlled ventilation).

Why do we use a log concentration–time curve?

Logging the concentration produces a straight line, which is mathematically much easier to work with than a curve (this graph is actually a semi-logarithmic plot because only the x-axis has been logged because time cannot be logged).

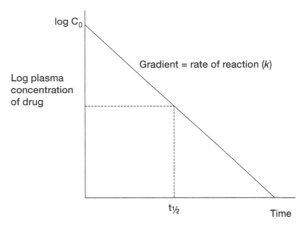

Fig. 10.2   Log of plasma drug concentration over time

What information can be derived from a log concentration–time curve?

> **Elimination rate constant (k)** is the rate of change in plasma concentration per unit time. It is the slope of the line.
> **Time constant (τ)** is the time it would take for the plasma concentration to reach zero had the original rate of change continued. It is the reciprocal of the elimination rate constant. It can be read directly from a concentration–time curve.
> **Plasma concentration at time zero (C_0)** can be read from the log concentration–time graph by extrapolating back onto the y-axis.

> **Half-life ($t_{1/2}$)** is the time taken for the plasma concentration to be reduced to half its original concentration. It can be read directly from the log concentration–time graph.

$$t_{1/2} = 0.693\tau \qquad or \qquad t_{1/2} = 0.693/k$$

> **Volume of distribution (V_D)** is the theoretical volume into which a drug must disperse in order to produce the measured plasma concentration.

$$V_D = Dose/C_0$$

> **Clearance (Cl)** is the volume of plasma completely cleared of a drug per unit time.

$$Cl = V_D \times k.$$

Simple Logarithmic Rules
- Logarithms are a way of expressing numbers as a power of a base.
- The base chosen most commonly is 10.
- So, the logarithm of a number is the power to which 10 would have to be raised to equal that number.

    E.g. log of 100 = 2   as 10^2 = 100 (10 × 10)
          log of 1000 = 3   as 10^3 = 1000 (10 × 10 × 10)

- We also use the 'natural logarithm', whose base is referred to as 'e'.
- e = 2.718 (approximately).
- So, the natural logarithm of number X is the power to which e would have to be raised to equal X.

When using logarithms:

- Multiplication becomes addition

    log (ab) = log (a) + log (b)

- Division becomes subtraction

    log (a/b) = log (a) – log (b)

- Power becomes multiplication

    log (a^b) = b.log(a)

- Reciprocal becomes negative

    log (1/a) = – log(a)

11. DOSE–RESPONSE CURVES

Draw a dose–response curve for a drug and explain its shape.

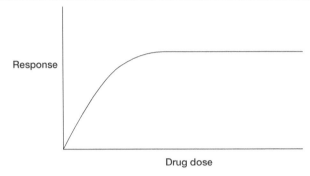

Response

Drug dose

Fig. 11.1 Dose–response curve

Initially, as the dose of drug increases, more receptors are stimulated, increasing the response. As the dose continues to increase, there are proportionally fewer receptors available for stimulation and, therefore, the response is proportionally less. Eventually, all the receptors are occupied and so an increase in dose does not affect an increase in response and the graph plateaus. This produces a rectangular hyperbola curve.

Why do we log the plot and what shape does this produce?

We log the dose to produce a sigmoid-shaped plot. It is easier and more accurate to extrapolate an estimated response to a given dose using this shape (as it is linear between 20% and 80% response), rather than the unlogged, rectangular hyperbola graph. It also allows us to predict the 'effective dose' of the drug, which will produce 50% and 95% of its maximal effect, the ED_{50} and ED_{95}.

> ED_{50} is the dose of a drug required to produce 50% of its maximal effect, or the dose of a drug that will produce a specified effect in 50% of the sample population.
> EC_{50} is the serum concentration of a drug required to produce 50% of its maximal effect, or the concentration of a drug that will produce a specified effect in 50% of the sample population.
> LD_{50} is the dose of a drug required to produce a lethal effect in 50% of the sample population.
> Therapeutic Ratio = LD_{50}/ED_{50}.

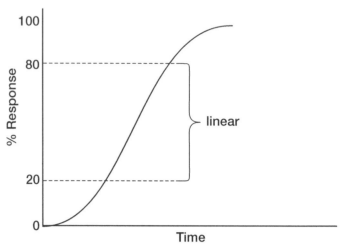

Fig. 11.2 Semi-logarithmic dose–response curve

Define the terms drug potency, affinity and efficacy.

> **Potency** describes the dose of drug required to produce a response of a given magnitude. A drug with a high potency requires a smaller dose than one of low potency to produce the same effect. Usually, the more lipid soluble a drug, the greater is its potency, e.g. fentanyl (1 µg/kg) is more potent than alfentanil (10 µg/kg).
> ED_{50} is used to define potency and compare drugs.
> **Affinity** describes how avidly a drug binds to its receptor. This is irrespective of whether the drug–receptor interaction produces a response or not.
> **Intrinsic activity** describes the extent to which the drug activates or stimulates a receptor once bound.
> **Efficacy** describes the ability of a drug to produce the maximal response or effect once it is bound to its receptor.

What do the following terms mean?

> **Full agonist**
  • Binds to receptors (has affinity) and produces a maximal response (efficacy = 1).
  • E.g. morphine acting on MOP receptors.
> **Partial agonist**
  • Binds to receptors (has affinity) but produces a sub-maximal response (efficacy <1).
  • E.g. buprenorphine acting on MOP receptors
> **Inverse agonist**
  • Bind to receptors (has affinity) but produces the opposite effect to the endogenous agonist (efficacy = –1).
  • E.g. naloxone acting on MOP receptors in morphine pre-treated tissues.
> **Antagonist**
  • Binds to receptors (has affinity) but exerts no effect of its own (efficacy = 0). Its presence inhibits the action of agonists of all types at that receptor.
  • E.g. atenolol acting on β adrenoceptors
> **Competitive antagonist**
  • Binds to receptors at the same site as the agonist and therefore competes with the agonist for this site. This antagonism can be overcome by increasing the concentration of the agonist.
  • E.g. vecuronium competing with ACh at nAChR.

> **Non-competitive antagonist**
  - Binds to receptors at a different site from the agonist and so does not prevent the agonist's binding to its receptor site. However, it alters the conformation of the receptor complex and prevents the agonist from eliciting a full response. Its effects are not overcome by increasing the agonist concentration.
  - E.g. ketamine acting at NMDA receptor.

> **Allosteric modulator**
  - Binds to the receptor at a site separate to that of the endogenous agonist. This alters the shape of the molecule, which either enhances or inhibits the affinity of the agonist for its receptor.
  - Allosteric modulators affect both affinity and efficacy of a drug, as opposed to competitive or non-competitive antagonists, which only alter one of these effects.
  - E.g. positive modulation: benzodiazepines increase the opening of the chloride channel at the $GABA_A$ receptor, which potentiates the effects of the inhibitory neurotransmitter GABA.
  - E.g. negative modulation: picrotoxin at the $GABA_A$ receptor.

Draw the log dose–response graph for an agonist in the presence of a competitive antagonist.

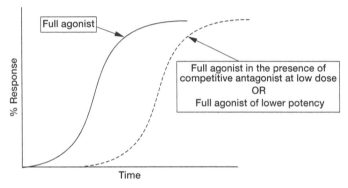

Fig. 11.3 Semi-logarithmic dose–response curve of an agonist in the presence of a competitive antagonist

Draw the log dose–response graph for an agonist in the presence of a non-competitive antagonist.

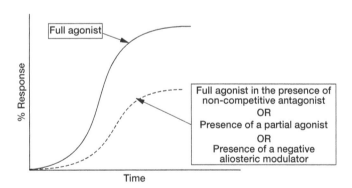

Fig. 11.4 Semi-logarithmic dose–response curve of an agonist in the presence of a non-competitive antagonist

What is the difference between tachyphylaxis and desensitisation?

> **Tachyphylaxis** is the acute reduction in response to a given dose after repeated administration of the drug.
>   • E.g. ephedrine (an indirectly acting sympathomimetic agent) will display tachyphylaxis due to depletion of presynaptic noradrenaline stores.
> **Desensitisation** is the chronic reduction in response to a given dose after repeated administration of the drug. This can be due to structural changes in the receptor and second messenger-dependent systems leading to altered drug affinity and impaired signal transduction processes. Receptor sequestration via endocytosis can also occur, leading to receptor down-regulation and loss of active receptors.
>   • E.g. dobutamine and adrenaline.

12. FIRST- AND ZERO-ORDER KINETICS

What are first-order kinetics?

> In first-order kinetics a **constant proportion** of the drug is eliminated from the body per unit time, e.g. 50% per hour and therefore clearance and half-life can be used to describe elimination kinetics.
> The **rate of elimination varies** and is directly proportional to the concentration of drug in the body at that time. This produces an exponential decay curve and is due to **non-saturable enzymes** being involved in drug elimination.
> The majority of drugs display first-order kinetics because the body contains more enzymes than needed to metabolise the clinically effective dose.

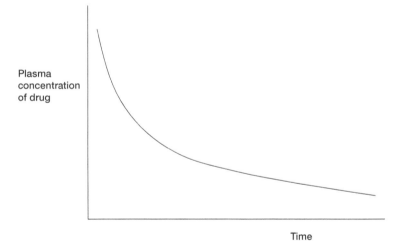

Plasma concentration of drug

Time

Fig. 12.1   First-order kinetics – plasma drug concentration over time

What are zero-order kinetics?

> In zero-order kinetics a **constant amount** of drug is eliminated from the body per unit time, e.g. 10 mg per hour and therefore clearance and half-life cannot be used to describe elimination kinetics.
> The **rate of elimination is constant** and changing the quantity of drug available for metabolism does not alter the rate of the reaction. This produces a linear graph because the **enzymes** involved in drug elimination become **saturated**.
> Ethanol, phenytoin, aspirin, theophylline and thiopentone display zero-order kinetics.

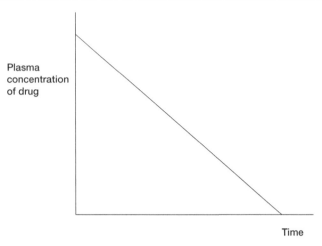

Fig. 12.2 Zero order kinetics-plasma drug concentration over time

Why is this important clinically?

> The therapeutic dose of some drugs is close to the plasma concentration at which the metabolic enzymes become saturated. Once saturated, a small increase in dosing or plasma drug concentration will result in greatly increased availability of the drug.
> If the drug has serious side effects, these too could become more pronounced. A common example of this is seen with alcohol intoxication, where consuming more than 1 unit/hour will lead to enzyme saturation, and the person concerned will become 'drunk'.

What are Michaelis–Menten kinetics?

> These describe the kinetics of the body's enzymes and are used to predict the rate of reaction between an enzyme (E) and substrate (S) to form a product (P).

$$S + E \rightleftharpoons ES \rightleftharpoons P$$

> In terms of drug elimination, E represents the enzymes involved in drug metabolism and S represents the plasma concentration of the drug.

Michaelis–Menten equation:

$$V = \frac{V_{max} \cdot [S]}{K_m + [S]}$$

Where:
V   velocity (or rate) of reaction
V$_{max}$ maximal rate of reaction
[S]   substrate (or drug) concentration
K$_m$ Michaelis constant, which is the substrate concentration at which $V = \frac{1}{2} V_{max}$

> At low substrate concentrations: $V \propto [S]$ – it obeys first-order kinetics and as the substrate concentration increases so does the rate of the reaction.
> At high substrate concentrations: $V \propto V_{max}$ – it obeys zero-order kinetics because the enzymes become saturated and the rate of reaction cannot increase any further.

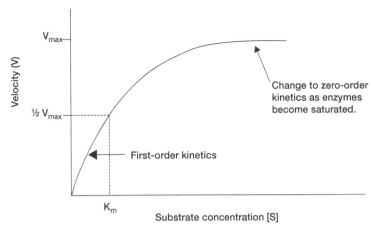

Fig. 12.3 Michaelis-Menten graph - velocity of reaction [V] over substrate concentration [S]

13. VOLUME OF DISTRIBUTION, CLEARANCE AND HALF-LIFE

Define volume of distribution.

> Volume of distribution (V_D) is the theoretical volume into which a drug must disperse in order to produce the measured plasma concentration.
> It cannot be measured directly but instead it is derived from a log concentration–time graph where $V_D = Dose/C_0$ (*see* Chapter 10, 'Exponential function').
> Its units are typically mL.

What factors determine the volume of distribution of a drug?

> Lipid solubility of the drug.
> Percentage plasma protein binding of the drug.
> Percentage tissue protein binding of the drug.
> Blood flow to the various tissues.

Define clearance.

> Clearance (Cl) is the volume of plasma completely cleared of a substance per unit time.
> It is usually constant over the therapeutic concentration range because drug elimination systems are not saturated (i.e. first-order kinetics).
> It is additive, a function of elimination by all participating organs such as liver or kidney: Cl systemic = $Cl_{renal} + Cl_{hepatic} + Cl_{other}$.
> Kidney and liver are the two most important sites for drug elimination, but other sites can include the lungs, muscle and plasma.
> It can be derived from a concentration–time graph where **Cl = Dose/AUC** (AUC = area under curve).
> Other equations used to calculate clearance include:
> • **Cl = rate of elimination/plasma concentration**
> • **Cl = $V_D \times k$**
> • **Cl = $V_D \times (0.693/t_{1/2})$**   (where 0.693 = ln2)
> It is used to describe elimination in first-order kinetics.
> Its units are typically mL/min.

Define half-life.

> Half-life ($t_{1/2}$) is the time taken for the plasma concentration of a substance to reduce to half its original value.
> It can be derived from a concentration–time graph.
> Equations used to calculate $t_{1/2}$ include:
> • **$t_{1/2} = 0.693 \times V_D/Cl$**
> • **$t_{1/2} = 0.693/k$**
> • **$t_{1/2} = 0.693\tau$**
> After five half-lives, elimination is 96.875% complete. Steady-state conditions are typically quoted to occur after five half-lives (or three time constants).
> Used to calculate dosing schedules.
> Its units are typically minutes (min).

How are V_D, Cl and $t_{1/2}$ interrelated?	$V_D \propto t_{1/2} \times Cl$ $\qquad t_{1/2} \propto V_D/Cl$ $\qquad Cl \propto V_D/t_{1/2}$

How can V_D, Cl and $t_{1/2}$ be used to explain the different clinical effects of fentanyl and alfentanil?

> Fentanyl is significantly more lipid soluble than alfentanil (i.e. more potent) and is therefore used in much smaller doses.
> Being more lipid soluble also accounts for the higher V_D of fentanyl because the drug can better penetrate tissues.
> The differences in the onset of effect can be explained by the pK_a values. Both fentanyl and alfentanil are basic compounds, which means that they become increasingly ionised below their pK_a. At physiological pH 7.35 (which is above the pK_a of alfentanil) 90% of alfentanil is in the un-ionised form and can therefore penetrate tissues easily to produce a rapid effect. For fentanyl, physiological pH is below its pK_a and therefore the majority of this drug gets ionised such that only 9% remains in the un-ionised form and this explains its longer onset of effect.
> The clearance of alfentanil is a lot slower than that of fentanyl but despite this it has a shorter duration of action because its smaller V_D ensures a shorter $t_{1/2}$.

Table 13.1 Pharmacokinetic comparison of fentanyl and alfentanil

Drug	Fentanyl	Alfentanil
Dose (µg/kg)	1	10
Onset (min)	5	1–2
Duration of action (min)	30	10
Lipid solubility	+++	+
pK_a	8.4	6.4
Percentage un-ionised	9	90
V_D (L/kg)	4	0.8
Cl (mL/min)	500–1500	300–500
$t_{1/2}$ (min)	360	120

14. COMPARTMENT MODELS

What is meant by the terms one-, two- and three-compartment models?

Compartment models are used to design mathematical models that will predict the drug-handling characteristics of the body. They help us calculate the doses and frequency of drug administration, and form the basis of anaesthetic infusion regimes used in target-controlled infusions.

One-compartment model
> The body is viewed as a single central compartment (C_1) with a defined volume of distribution.
> When a drug is administered (rate constant k_{01}) it is assumed to disperse instantaneously and uniformly throughout C_1.
> It is also assumed that the drug is then completely cleared from C_1 by elimination alone (rate constant k_{10}).
> This model produces a mono-exponential decay curve.
> Semi-logarithmic plot produces a straight line.
> In reality, this model is far too simplistic because plasma drug concentrations decline due to a multitude of factors including distribution from plasma into different tissues (which can occur at different rates due to differences in tissue perfusion), drug metabolism and excretion. Therefore a less simplistic model with two or three compartments is required.

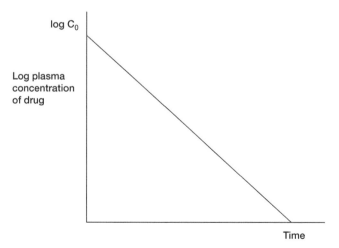

Fig. 14.1   Semi-logarithmic plot of plasma concentration of drug over time

Two-compartment model

> The body is now viewed as a central compartment (C_1 – representing plasma) in conjunction with a peripheral compartment (C_2 – representing tissues).
> Additional rate constants apply to this model and plasma drug concentrations now decline due to drug distribution from plasma to tissues (k_{12}) and drug elimination from the central compartment (k_{10}).
> This produces a bi-phasic exponential decay curve.

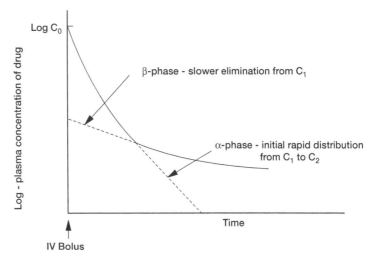

Fig. 14.2 Semi-logarithmic plot showing bi-exponential decay of plasma concentration of drug over time in a two-compartment model

Three-compartment model

> The body is viewed as a central compartment (C_1 – representing plasma), an intermediately well-perfused peripheral compartment (C_2 – representing tissues like muscle) and a poorly perfused peripheral compartment (C_3 – representing tissues like fat).
> Additional rate constants apply to this model and plasma drug concentrations now decline due to drug distribution into the peripheral compartments of C_2 (k_{12}) and C_3 (k_{13}) and drug elimination from the central compartment (k_{10}).
> This produces a tri-phasic exponential decay curve where the distribution part of the curve can be divided into a fast (α) and slow (β) phase followed by an elimination phase.
> The distribution to and redistribution from the peripheral compartments along with drug elimination from the central compartment occurs simultaneously and down concentration gradients.
> Peripheral compartments can act as stores for the drug, keeping the central compartment full even after drug administration into it has ceased and drug elimination from it continues.
> This redistribution of drug into the central explains why the effect of a drug can continue long after its administration has ended and this is an integral concept in target-controlled infusions and context-sensitive half-lives (*see* Chapter 15, 'Total intravenous anaesthesia').

15. TOTAL INTRAVENOUS ANAESTHESIA

What is meant by the term 'total intravenous anaesthesia'?

> Total intravenous anaesthesia (TIVA) refers to anaesthesia that is provided solely by the intravenous route, e.g. propofol infusion.
> It is generally administered as a continuous infusion. This infusion can be either run at a specific rate or titrated to achieve a specific concentration of the agent, either in the plasma (C_p), or at the brain, i.e. the effect site (C_e), by running a 'target-controlled' infusion.

What are the indications for using TIVA?

> When inhalational agents are not available, e.g. ITU, transfers and field anaesthesia.
> When administering inhalational agents is difficult, e.g. during bronchoscopy.
> When inhalational agents are contraindicated, e.g. malignant hyperpyrexia.
> To reduce post-operative nausea and vomiting.
> To reduce exposure of staff to inhalational agents.
> To reduce pollution.

What are the properties of an ideal intravenous anaesthetic agent?

> Ideal physical properties:
>   • Cheap
>   • Stable and non-reactive with plastics, glass and metal
>   • Long shelf life
>   • Water soluble and so easy to formulate and store
>   • Environmentally safe
> Ideal pharmacokinetic properties:
>   • Rapid onset and offset, i.e. lipid soluble
>   • Minimal accumulation in body tissues, i.e. small V_D
>   • Rapid metabolism in plasma to inactive products giving a context 'insensitive' half-time
>   • No excitation or emergence phenomena
>   • No interaction with other drugs
> Ideal pharmacodynamic properties:
>   • Painless on injection
>   • Analgesic, muscle relaxant and antiemetic
>   • No effect on patient's physiology
>   • No toxic effect
>   • No hypersensitivity reactions or histamine release

What is meant by the term 'target-controlled infusion'?

> Target-controlled infusion (TCI) refers to an infusion system where the target concentration of the agent in the plasma or the effect site can be chosen.

What are the pharmacokinetic principles used in designing a TCI?	> TCI designs are based on pharmacokinetic mathematical models like the three-compartment model (*see* Chapter 14, 'Compartment models').
	> Pharmacokinetic data sets for the infused drug are incorporated into this mathematical model (e.g. V_D, Cl, $t_{1/2}$, k).
	> Patient data, e.g. age, weight, height and sex, are also entered into the model.
	> The mathematical model then predicts the plasma and effect site concentration of the drug and adjusts the infusion rate according to these predictions.
What are the limitations of such a pharmacokinetic mathematical model?	> These models are based on several assumptions as follows:
	> Tissues only have either a high or a low blood flow with specific rate constants for distribution, redistribution and clearance.
	> All people have the same proportion of different tissues.
	> All people metabolise and eliminate the drug at the same rate.
	> All people will become anaesthetised at the same target concentration.
	> There is no in vivo measurement of the actual plasma or effect site concentration of the drug. The data produced are merely predictions based on mathematical models, pharmacokinetic data sets and normograms.
What is context-sensitive half-time?	> Context-sensitive half-time (CSHT) is applicable to intravenous infusions of drugs. It is the time taken for the drug concentration to reduce by half once an infusion designed to maintain a constant plasma concentration is stopped.
	> The term 'context' refers to the duration of drug infusion prior to stopping.
	> CSHT for a specific drug will vary depending on the duration of the infusion.
What causes context-sensitive half-times?	> During an infusion, the plasma will have the highest concentration of the drug in the body and therefore the drug will tend to travel down its concentration gradient into various tissues until tissue and plasma concentrations reach equilibrium.
	> If the infusion is given for long enough for plasma concentration to reach equilibrium with the tissues, there will be no net movement of the drug between compartments as long as the rate of infusion matches the rate of elimination of the drug.
	> Tissues with a high perfusion will equilibrate with plasma faster than those with low perfusion. Tissues with a high fat content and poor perfusion will act as a store.
	> Once a drug infusion has stopped, the drug concentration in the plasma will start to fall as the drug is metabolised and excreted.
	> The tissues will then have a higher concentration of the drug compared with the plasma and hence drug will redistribute from these tissues into the plasma.
	> The longer the duration of an infusion, the more drug will accumulate in the tissues, forming a store that can then replenish and maintain the plasma levels as the drug is metabolised and excreted.
	> This results in the context-sensitive half-life.

Which drugs lend themselves well to infusion regimes?

> Drugs with a small volume of distribution, rapid metabolism (with no active metabolites), high clearance and short CSHT are ideal for infusions.
> Remifentanil, propofol and alfentanil are the three main anaesthetic agents used in TCI.

Table 15.1 Context-sensitive half-times for various agents

Drug	CSHT after 2-h infusion	CSHT after 8-h infusion
Remifentanil	4.5 min	9 min
Propofol	16 min	41 min
Alfentanil	50 min	64 min
Fentanyl	48 min	282 min

Draw a graph showing the context-sensitive half-times of commonly infused drugs.

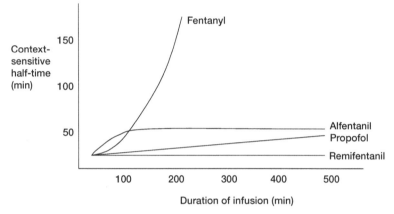

Fig. 15.1 Comparison of effect of duration of infusion on context-sensitive half-times for various agents

What is unique about remifentanil infusion?

> Remifentanil is rapidly broken down by non-specific plasma and tissue esterases.
> It has a short elimination half-time ($t_{1/2}$ = 1.3 min), high clearance (2.5 L/kg/h) and small volume of distribution (0.35 L/kg), giving it a relatively constant context-sensitive half-time of 3–10 minutes.
> Remifentanil is therefore often said to have a context-'insensitive' half-time.

16. INDUCTION AGENTS

A complete knowledge of the common induction agents will be expected. This will include the class of drug, mechanism of action (where known), presentation, uses, dose, systemic effects, side effects, pharmacokinetics and interactions.

The required information for each induction agent is presented in the form of spider diagrams, which allow easy comparison of the drugs. Keep in mind the properties of an ideal induction agent:

Physical properties:
> Cheap and easy to make
> Long shelf life at room temperature
> Water soluble and so easy to store
> Painless on injection
> Safe if injected intra-arterially
> Rapid onset time
> Rapid offset time
> No excitation or emergence phenomena
> No accumulation following infusion
> No interaction with other drugs

Biological properties:
> Analgesic
> No effects on patient's physiology, other than rendering them unconscious
> No toxic effects

Propofol

USES
- Induction and maintenance of anaesthesia
- Sedation
- Refractory nausea and vomiting
- Status epilepticus

ABSORPTION/ DISTRIBUTION
- Protein binding 98%
- V_D 4 L/kg
- Rapid distribution to tissues
- Rapid elimination ($t_{1/2}$ 1–5 hours, context sensitive) which may be increased following slower release from adipose tissue

MOA
- Uncertain
- May potentiate $GABA_A$ receptor
- May have action at cannabinoid receptor

EFFECTS
CVS
- $\downarrow$BP and SV (15%–25%)
- $\downarrow$CO (25%)
- Vasodilatation secondary to NO production
- Bradycardia/ asystole
RS
- Depression
- $\downarrow$Laryngeal reflex
- $\uparrow$RR$\downarrow$$V_T$
- $\downarrow$Response to$\uparrow$$pCO_2$ and $\downarrow$$pO_2$
- Bronchodilation
CNS
- Hypnotic, smooth and rapid induction $\downarrow$ CPP$\downarrow$ICP$\downarrow$$CMRO_2$
- Myoclonic movements
GI
- Antiemetic (antagonist at D_2 receptor)
SIDE-EFFECTS
- Pain on injection (improved with newer 'Propfol-Lipura®' which has $\uparrow$medium chain triglycerides rendering drug more lipid-soluble)
- Epileptiform movements (however it is not epileptogenic and is used for treatment of status epileptious)
- Unlicensed in $\leq$16 yr olds after complications of long-term use in ICU (fat overload syndrome, fatty deposits in liver, lung, heart and kidneys/metabolic acidosis/refractory bradycardia)
- Lipaemia with long-term use
- Green urine and hair, secondary to quinol metabolites
- Increased energy needed for DCCV
- Physically incompatible with atracurium

PROPOFOL
(2,6-diisopropylphenol)
Phenolic derivative
- 1%/2% white lipid-water emulsion in soya bean oil and purified egg phosphatide
- 20/50/100 mL vials and 50 mL pre-filled syringe

DOSE
- 1.5–2.5 mg/kg (adult)
- 2–7 mg/kg (child)
- 4–12 mcg/kg/hr maintenance

METABOLISM AND EXCRETION
- Hepatic metabolism, mainly conjugated to inactive glucuronide
- Renal excretion
- Liver/renal dysfunction has little effect on metabolism
- Clearance exceeds hepatic blood flow, suggestive of extra hepatic metabolism
- No active metabolites

CHEMICAL PROPERTIES
- Poorly water soluble
- Weak organic acid
- pK_a = 11 $\therefore$ almost totally un-ionised at pH 7.4
- pH 7.0
- Free radical scavenger
- Physically incompatible with atracurium

Thiopentone

USES
- Induction of anaesthesia (bolus lasts 5–10 min)
- Status epilepticus
- To achieve 'burst suppression' in raised ICP

ABSORPTION/ DISTRIBUTION
- Protein binding 80%
- Of the unbound 20%, only 12% un-ionised and available (as 60% ionised at pH 7.4)
- V_D 2 L/kg
- Rapid emergence secondary to rapid redistribution to tissues
- Critically ill patients are acidotic with ↓ protein binding ∴ less thiopentone needed
- NSAIDs may ↓ protein binding and ∴ ↑ free drug fraction

MOA
- ↑ Duration of opening of GABA Cl⁻ channels in CNS causes hyperpolarisation and neuronal inhibition

THIOPENTONE
Barbiturate
- Yellow powder, 500 mg/vial

DOSE
- 3–7 mg/kg IV
- 1 g/22 kg weight PR

EFFECTS
CVS
- ↓ CO
- ↓ SV
- ↓ SVR
- May cause ↑ HR
RS
- Depression
- Laryngospasm
- Bronchospasm
CNS
- Anaesthesia
- ↓ $CMRO_2$
- ↓ Blood flow and volume
- ↓ CSF pressure
- At low dose is antalgesic
RENAL
- ↓ Urine OP (↑ ADH and ↓ CO)
OTHER
- Severe anaphylaxis (1/20 000)
- Precipitates porphyria
- Intra-arterial injection → severe pain and spasm and perivascular necrosis

METABOLISM AND EXCRETION
- Hepatic oxidation by P450 → mainly inactive metabolites (though pentobarbitone is active)
- Induces P450 after single dose
- Zero order kinetics with infusion

CHEMICAL PROPERTIES
- Displays tautomerism or dynamic isomerism, the proportions of the two forms governed by ambient pH
- Weak acid – forms alkaline solution when dissolved in H_2O, pH 10.8. This solution stable for many days and is bacteriostatic because of high pH.
- Undissociated acid insoluble and so, when packaged:
  a) Sodium carbonate (6% by weight) added to powder. So, when dissolved, it releases –OH⁻, ∴ preventing accumulation of H^+ and formation of undissociated acid
  b) Stored under N_2 gas – prevents acidification of powder by CO_2 in air
- pK_a 7.6 ∴ 60% un-ionised at pH 7.4
- Highly lipid soluble

Etomidate

USES
- Induction of anaesthesia
- Treatment of Cushing's syndrome before surgery

MOA
- ↑ Duration of opening of GABA Cl⁻ channels in CNS causes hyperpolarisation and neuronal inhibition
- Only the D isomer causes hypnosis

ABSORPTION/ DISTRIBUTION
- Protein binding 75%
- Rapid distribution
- V_D 3 L/kg

ETOMIDATE
Imidazole hypnotic
- Clear colourless solution: 2 mg/mL in 10 mL vial

DOSE
- 0.3 mg/kg

METABOLISM AND EXCRETION
- Rapid metabolism by hepatic and plasma esterases
- May inhibit plasma cholinesterase
- Excreted in urine (90%) and bile (10%)

CHEMICAL PROPERTIES
- pH of solution 8.1
- pk_a 4.1

EFFECTS
CVS
- Most stable induction agent
- Slight ↓ SVR
- Myocardial O_2 consumption not affected
- Contractility not affected
- BP not affected

RS
- Depression
- No inhibition of hypoxic pulmonary vasoconstriction

CNS
- Hypnosis
- Tremor
- Involuntary movements
- ↓ Tone
- Epileptiform activity on EEG in 25%
- ↓ ICP
- ↓ CPP and ↓CMRO$_2$
- ↓ IOP

GI
- Nausea and vomiting (especially in conjunction with opioid)

OTHER
- Inhibits steroid synthesis, by inhibition of 11β and 17α-hydroxylase, for 24 hourly after only 1 dose. Was associated with deaths on ICU following infusion for sedation. Use has declined because of this and the increasing popularity of ketamine
- Pain on injection in 25%
- Contraindicated in porphyria
- Antiplatelet activity
- Hypersensitivity and histamine release (rare)

Ketamine

USES
- Induction and maintenance of anaesthesia especially in refractory asthma because of its profound bronchodilator effects
- Sedation on ICU/for short procedures, e.g. dressing change in burns
- Analgesia especially in the military field
- In neuroaxial blockade to prolong its effect
- Drug of abuse

ABSORPTION/ DISTRIBUTION
- Well absorbed orally and IM
- Oral bioavailability 20%
- Protein binding 20–50%
- V_D 3 L/kg
- $t_{1/2}$ 2.5 hours

MOA
- Non-competitive antagonist at NMDA receptor
- Weak agonist at MOP KOP and DOP receptors
- Inhibits reuptake of serotonin, dopamine and noradrenaline

EFFECTS
CVS
- ↑ noradrenaline and adrenaline release
- ↑ HR
- ↑ CO
- ↑ BP
- ↑ Cardiac O_2 consumption

RS
- ↑ RR
- No ↓ laryngeal reflex
- Airway maintained
- Profound bronchodilation

CNS
- Dissociative anaesthesia (i.e. strong analgesic and light 'sleep')
- ↑CBF/ ↑ICP/ ↑CMRO$_2$
- Traditionally avoided in head injury as it was thought to ↑ ICP. In fact it does this no more than opioios do.
- ↑ IOP
- Amnesia
- Emergence phenomena, delirium, hallucinations. Reduced by co-administration of benzodiazepine
- ↑ Muscle tone

GI
- Nauea and vomiting
- Salivation

KETAMINE
Phencyclidine derivative
- Colourless solution in glass vial: 10/50/100 mg/mL
- Available as racemic mix or as S (+) enantiomer (less delirium)
- IV/IM/PO/PR/intrathecal/ epidural administration
- Induction dose: 1–2 mg/kg IV 5–10 mg/kg IM
- Analgesic dose: 0.2–0.5 mg/kg

METABOLISM AND EXCRETION
- Metabolised in liver by P450 to norketamine (30% potency)
- Norketamine metabolised by conjugation to inactive compound
- Excreted in urine

CHEMICAL PROPERTIES
- Chiral compound most preparations are racemic, but S-Ketamine is available as single enantiomer
- S-Ketamine is twice as potent as racemic mixture
- Inhibits dopamine transporters 8x more than R-Ketamine
- 3-4x affinity for NMDA receptor than R-Ketamine
- Patients report more pleasant experience at doses causing same effect
- Recover mental function more quickly
- Water soluble forming acidic solution pH 3.5–5.5

17. NITROUS OXIDE

The use of nitrous oxide (N_2O) is declining in UK anaesthetic practice. However, it remains widely available and examiners will expect a balanced answer illustrating the advantages and disadvantages of N_2O use.

How is nitrous oxide produced?

Ammonium nitrate is heated to 250 °C causing it to decompose:

$$NH_4NO_3 \longrightarrow N_2O + 2H_2O$$

If temperature is not controlled carefully during production, contaminants may accumulate in the gas (e.g. NH_3, N_2, NO, NO_2 and HNO_3). Any impurities are removed prior to storage.

How is nitrous oxide stored?

> N_2O is stored in cylinders coloured 'French blue'.
> It is stored as a liquid, below its critical temperature (36.5 °C)

List the physicochemical properties of N_2O.

> Boiling point –88 °C
> Critical temperature 36.5 °C
> Critical pressure 72 bar
> Blood/gas partition coefficient 0.47
> Oil/gas partition coefficient 1.4
> MAC 105% (only under hyperbaric conditions can N_2O produce full anaesthesia)

List its pharmacodynamic properties.

Cardiovascular:
> Reduces myocardial contractility but increases sympathetic outflow, resulting in a minimal change in blood pressure.
> Increases pulmonary vascular resistance and should be avoided in patients with known pulmonary hypertension.

Respiratory:
> Causes a reduction in tidal volume and an increase in respiratory rate, resulting in maintenance of minute ventilation.
> Blunts the ventilatory responses to both hypoxia and hypercarbia.

Neurological:
> Increases cerebral blood flow, cerebral metabolic requirement for oxygen and intracranial pressure.
> Effects are more pronounced in patients with loss of cerebral autoregulation, e.g. traumatic brain injury.

How is N_2O used clinically?

General anaesthesia:
> As a carrier gas.
> To reduce the amount of volatile agent used because of its MAC-sparing effect (e.g. 0.5 MAC N_2O + 0.5 MAC sevoflurane = 1 MAC). This is due to its inhibitory action at NMDA (glutamate) receptors and agonist activity at dopamine receptors.
> To give faster onset of inhalational anaesthesia using the 'concentration effect' and the 'second gas effect'. N_2O is 30 times more soluble in blood than nitrogen and therefore diffuses more rapidly across the alveolar membrane into the blood than nitrogen can diffuse out into the alveoli. This results in reduced alveolar volume and a rise in alveolar partial pressure and concentration of the remaining gases. This is the 'concentration effect'. Because the concentration gradient of volatile agent between alveoli and blood is now increased, there is faster diffusion of volatile agents into the blood and therefore faster onset of anaesthesia. This is the 'second gas effect'.

Analgesia:
> N_2O is a good analgesic, exhibiting agonist activity at opioid receptors and acting at a spinal cord level through modulation of descending noradrenergic pain pathways.
> It is mixed with oxygen to form Entonox (50% O_2 and 50% N_2O), which is used for pain relief, predominantly during labour.

What are its adverse effects?

Post-operative nausea and vomiting (PONV):
> The use of N_2O during general anaesthesia is associated with an increased incidence of PONV. The exact aetiology is unclear but may involve bowel distension, middle ear or opioid effects.

Expansion of nitrogen-containing cavities:
> This occurs because N_2O is more soluble than nitrogen and so it diffuses from the blood into air-filled cavities more quickly than nitrogen already in the cavity can diffuse back into the blood.
> Use of N_2O results in increased pressure in air-filled spaces, e.g. middle ear, pneumothoraces, endotracheal cuffs (during prolonged surgery) and bowel. It is therefore contraindicated in certain types of surgery.

Bone marrow toxicity and CNS toxicity:
> N_2O oxidises the cobalt ion in the vitamin B_{12} complex, impairing its ability to act as a co-factor for the enzyme methionine synthase.
> This causes bone marrow suppression and therefore reduced DNA, methionine, thymidine and tetrahydrofolate synthesis. The result is megaloblastic anaemia and subacute degeneration of the spinal cord (dorsal columns) leading to neuropathy.

Teratogenicity:
> Has occurred in rats, but never in humans.
> The exact mechanism is likely to be multi-factorial, but includes impaired DNA synthesis and α_1-adrenoceptor agonist activity, which is associated with situs inversus.

Environmental pollutant:
> N_2O is a greenhouse gas; however, anaesthetic emissions account for a tiny proportion of total nitrous oxide emissions, especially with low-flow anaesthesia.

Describe some properties of Entonox.

Entonox is the trade name for the mixture 50:50 $N_2O:O_2$.

> It is stored as a gas in cylinders with a French blue body and blue and white striped shoulders.
> A full cylinder has a pressure of 137 bar.
> When the N_2O and O_2 dissolve into each other, the resulting gas takes on properties unpredictable from its constituents. This is called the 'Poynting effect'.
> The pseudocritical temperature of the mixture is −7 °C. Below this temperature the N_2O will convert to its liquid phase, in a process called lamination. Anyone using this cylinder will receive only O_2, followed by a mixture of O_2 and N_2O, and finally only the hypoxic N_2O. If Entonox has been stored below its pseudocritical temperature, the cylinder should be warmed and inverted several times to ensure mixing before use.

18. INHALATIONAL ANAESTHETIC AGENTS (VOLATILE AGENTS)

Explain the terms 'blood:gas' and 'oil:gas' partition coefficient differences.

A partition coefficient is the ratio of the amount of substance in one phase to the amount of it in another at a stated temperature, when the two phases are in equilibrium and of equal volumes and pressures.

At a steady state, the partial pressure of volatile anaesthetic agents within the alveoli (P_A) is in equilibrium with that in the arterial blood (P_a) and subsequently the brain (P_B). As such, P_A gives an indirect measure of P_B.

The blood:gas (B:G) coefficient is a measure of the solubility of a substance in blood and influences anaesthetic onset and offset times.

> The more soluble an inhalational agent, the slower its onset and offset times. This is because its effects on the central nervous system depend on its partial pressure in blood (and subsequently its partial pressure in the brain) and not on the absolute amount dissolved in blood.
> Highly soluble agents (halothane and isoflurane) have low partial pressures in blood and more molecules are required to saturate the liquid phase before the P_A can be increased.
> As the molecules within the alveoli are readily taken up into the blood, the alveolar concentration and partial pressure remain low, and it takes longer to reach equilibrium (F_A/F_i ratio of 1).
> Consequently, the brain partial pressure rises more slowly and the onset of anaesthesia is slower.
> Conversely, poorly soluble agents (desflurane and sevoflurane) have alveolar concentrations that rise rapidly towards inspired concentrations, achieving higher partial pressures in alveoli, blood and brain, and onset of anaesthesia is more rapid.

The wash-in curves (F_A/F_i ratio over time) graphically demonstrate the effect of B:G coefficients on onset times for different agents. F_A/F_i represents the ratio of fractional alveolar to fractional inspired concentrations, and different agents achieve an F_A/F_i ratio of 1 (equilibrium) at different rates.

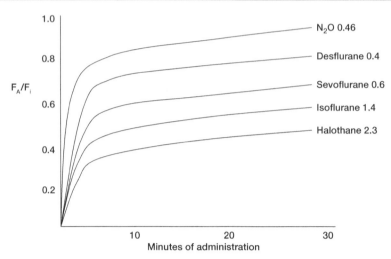

Fig. 18.1 Wash in curves showing the inspired concentration of inhalational agent (F$_i$) against alveolar concentration (F$_A$) over time

The oil:gas (O:G) coefficient is a measure of lipid solubility and an indicator of potency. It is inversely related to MAC.

> Highly lipid-soluble agents are more potent and a lower MAC is required to achieve central nervous system effects.
> The Meyer–Overton theory (*see* p. 57) suggests that when sufficient amount of agent dissolves into a neuronal lipid membrane, anaesthesia is achieved. Using logarithmic scales, MAC can be plotted against O:G for various agents. If this hypothesis were correct, then the product of MAC and O:G would be a single constant. In fact, for the older agents, the product equates to 100, whereas for the newer agents, it equals 200, suggesting there may be different sites or mechanisms of action.

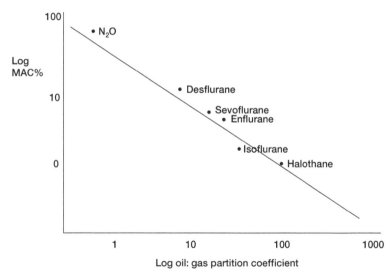

Fig. 18.2 The relationship between MAC and lipid solubility

Compare the uptake and excretion of isoflurane and sevoflurane.

Table 18.1 Physiochemical properties of isoflurane compared to sevoflurane

Property	Isoflurane	Sevoflurane
Blood:Gas coefficient	1.4	0.6
Onset/offset	Slower	Faster
Oil:Gas coefficient	98	53
MAC (in 100% O_2)	1.15	2.05
MAC (in 70% N_2O)	0.56	0.66
Metabolism (%)	0.2	3–5

Isoflurane is more soluble in blood and exerts a lower partial pressure in blood. As it easily diffuses out of the alveoli, it takes longer than sevoflurane to achieve a high alveolar partial pressure. Consequently its ratio of alveolar concentration to inspired concentration (F_A/F_I) takes longer to approach 1 and its speed of onset of anaesthesia is slower. The converse applies at the end of anaesthesia when the offset time of isoflurane is slower.

Which factors, other than blood:gas coefficient, affect the speed of onset of anaesthesia when using volatiles?

The increase in alveolar partial pressure (P_A) is a balance between the delivery of the drug to the alveolus and the loss from the alveolus to the arterial blood (input minus uptake).

> **Inspired concentration (F_I):** If high, there is an increased delivery of drug to the alveolus and a more rapid rise in P_A. In turn, F_I depends on the:
>   • Concentration set on the vaporiser
>   • Fresh gas flow rate
>   • Volume of the breathing circuit
>   • Amount absorbed by the anaesthetic machine and breathing circuit.
> **Alveolar minute ventilation:** If high, the delivery of volatile agent to the alveolus is increased. In turn, this is influenced by:
>   • Respiratory depressant effects of the volatile agents with increasing depth of anaesthesia as hypocapnia causes a reduced cerebral blood flow and reduced delivery of agent to the brain
>   • Ventilatory settings in ventilated patients.
> **Functional residual capacity (FRC):** A large FRC will dilute the inspired concentration, resulting in a slower rise in P_A and a slower onset, whereas a small FRC leads to a rapid rise in P_A and a faster onset.
> **Cardiac output and pulmonary blood flow:** If high, the agent is taken up from the alveolus more effectively and so the P_A rises more slowly, leading to a slower onset of anaesthesia. A low cardiac output results in a slower uptake into the circulation, achieving a higher P_A more quickly. The onset of anaesthesia is more rapid. The myocardial depressant effects of volatile agents thus have a positive feedback effect on their onset.
> **$\dot{V}/\dot{Q}$ mismatch and diffusion defects:** These are rarely significant.
> **Concentration and second gas effect:** The concentration effect occurs when N_2O is used in high concentration and refers to the disproportionate rise in alveolar partial pressures of other gases. N_2O is much more soluble than N_2 (35×) and O_2 (20×) and results in a reduced alveolar volume as it diffuses out of the alveoli more rapidly than N_2 can diffuse back in. The reduced alveolar volume results in a rise in alveolar partial pressure and concentration of the remaining gases.

The second gas effect refers to the effect that N_2O has on the speed of onset of anaesthesia of the second gas (volatile). As a consequence of the concentration effect, the volatile agents achieve a rapid rise in P_A, and their F_A/F_I ratio approaches 1 more quickly, leading to a faster onset of action.

The same factors will affect the speed of offset (elimination) of inhalational anaesthetic agents.

How does the structure of an inhalational agent influence its effects?

> All volatile agents, except halothane and nitrous oxide, are halogenated ethers.
> An ether is a link between two carbon-containing compounds (C–O–C).
> Ethers are lipid soluble but not water soluble.
> A halogen is a member of group VII of the periodic table, which includes fluorine (F), chlorine (Cl) and bromine (Br).
> Fluorine is the lightest of the three and lowers the molecular weight (MW) of the compound. A lower MW increases blood solubility, and a higher MW increases potency. Fluorine is the most electronegative halogen and stabilises ethers. It increases the saturated vapour pressure and therefore the compound evaporates less easily (e.g. desflurane).
> Halothane is a halogen-substituted alkane (halogenated hydrocarbon). An alkane is a hydrocarbon with fully saturated bonds, such as methane (CH_4) and ethane (CH_3CH_3). Alkanes are lipid soluble and precipitate arrhythmias.
> Halogenation reduces flammability.
> Halothane is a halogen-substituted alkane (MW = 197).
> Isoflurane is a halogenated methyl ethyl ether (MW = 184).
> Enflurane is a halogenated methyl ethyl ether (MW = 184). Isoflurane and enflurane are structural isomers.
> Desflurane is a fluorinated methyl ethyl ether (MW = 168).
> Sevoflurane is a polyfluorinated isopropyl methyl ether (MW = 200).
> Nitrous oxide exists in two forms as a hybrid.

What are the harmful effects of inhalational anaesthetic agents?

> **Hepato- and nephrotoxicity**
  Inhaled anaesthetic agents undergo metabolism in the liver via cytochrome P450 system. The carbon–halogen bond releases the halogen ion, which is potentially nephrotoxic. The C–F bond is more stable and minimally metabolised, whereas the C–Cl and C–Br bonds are more easily metabolised. Inorganic fluoride ions may be nephrotoxic.
> **Bone marrow depression**
  Nitrous oxide is only minimally metabolised (0.004%) by gut organisms. Nitrous oxide oxidises the cobalt atom in vitamin B_{12} complex, which acts as a co-factor for the enzyme methionine synthetase. The resultant bone marrow depression may be apparent by the development of:
  • Subacute degeneration of the spinal cord (dorsal columns) due to inhibition of methionine synthesis.
  • Megaloblastic anaemia due to impaired tetrahydrofolate production (important substrate in DNA synthesis).
> **Compound A**
  Sevoflurane administered via a circle system can react with soda and baralyme used to absorb CO_2, resulting in the production of compounds A, B, C, D and E. Only A is potentially toxic (kidneys, brain, liver), but in clinical practice, the concentrations produced are much lower than the toxic threshold (200 ppm).
> **Halothane hepatitis**
  This is thought to manifest in one of two ways:
  • Reversible transaminitis due to hepatic hypoxia
  • Fulminant hepatitis, which is an antigen–antibody reaction. The metabolite trifluoroacetic acid combines with liver proteins (haptens), stimulating the production of antibodies to hapten, and precipitating hepatic necrosis. Risk factors include repeated exposure, female sex, obesity and middle age. Mortality is 50–70%. In theory, it may occur with other agents, but their low rates of metabolism make this less likely.

Table 18.2 Metabolic products of commonly used inhalational agents

Agent	% Metabolism	Metabolite
N_2O	<0.01	N_2
Halothane	20	Trifluoroacetic acid, chloride and bromide ions
Enflurane	2	Inorganic and organic fluorides
Isoflurane	0.2	Trifluoroacetic acid fluoride ions
Sevoflurane	3–5	Inorganic and organic fluorides Compounds A, B, C, D, E
Desflurane	0.02	Trifluoroacetic acid

How do inhalational anaesthetic agents exert their effects?

Different hypotheses have been put forward, but no single hypothesis adequately explains their effects.

> **Meyer–Overton hypothesis:** This was put forward 100 years ago and describes a link between lipid solubility (oil:gas coefficient) and potency (MAC). The critical volume hypothesis expands on this theory and states that when sufficient amounts of inhalational agents dissolve into the neuronal lipid membrane, ion channels become distorted and synaptic transmission is impaired. The effect of combined inhalational agents is additive.

> **Membrane protein receptor hypothesis:** Binding sites for anaesthetic agents on transmembrane proteins have been found. Many ion channels or receptors are likely to be involved including acetylcholine, $GABA_A$, NMDA and voltage-gated ion channels.

> **Alteration in neurotransmitter availability and action on receptors:** The breakdown of the inhibitory neurotransmitter gamma amino butyric acid (GABA) is inhibited by volatile agents, leading to an accumulation of GABA within the central nervous system and activation of the $GABA_A$ receptor, causing hyperpolarisation of the cell membrane. Volatile agents may inhibit certain calcium channels, preventing the release of neurotransmitters, and may inhibit the glutamate receptor.

> **Multi-site hypothesis:** Different inhalational agents alter higher central nervous system function (memory, learning and consciousness) at different concentrations. Furthermore, certain agents, e.g. opiates, may reduce MAC, although this effect is neither predictable nor additive. This implies that there are different sites of action and that inhaled anaesthetics may have both a direct and an indirect effect (via second messengers) on ion channels at various concentrations.

Which neurotransmitters are implicated in the mode of action of inhalational anaesthetic agents?

> **Excitatory** neurotransmitters, e.g. glutamate and acetylcholine, are thought to be inhibited.

> **Inhibitory neurotransmitters**, e.g. GABA and glycine, are thought to be activated.

> Nitrous oxide does not appear to affect the $GABA_A$ receptor but strongly inhibits the NMDA receptor. It stimulates dopaminergic neurones, mediating the release of endogenous opioids.

What effects do isoflurane, sevoflurane and desflurane have on the cardiovascular system?

All the halogenated agents cause dose-dependent cardiovascular depression with varying effects.

Table 18.3 Comparison of the cardiovascular effects of isoflurane, sevoflurane and desflurane

	Isoflurane	Sevoflurane	Desflurane
SVR	↓↓	↓	↓ above 2.2 MAC
MAP	↓	↓	↓
HR	↑↑	↓	↑↑
CO	↔	↔	↔
Contractility	↔ initially ↓ at high doses	↔ initially ↓ at high doses	↔ initially ↓ (less than other agents)
Myocardial work & O_2 consumption	↓	↓↓	↓
Dysrhythmogenic	No	No	No
Coronary steal	Yes	Possible	Possible

What is MAC?

> MAC is the minimum alveolar concentration, at equilibrium (15 minutes of inhalation), at sea level, in 100% oxygen, at which 50% of the population will fail to respond to a standard noxious stimulus. This is MAC_{50} and is the standard accepted MAC. The stimulus refers to a standard surgical skin incision, and the response refers to purposeful muscular movement.
> MAC_{90} is the concentration required to prevent movement in 90% of subjects.
> It is a measure of potency and allows comparison between different agents.
> MAC is additive when inhalational agents are administered simultaneously.
> MAC awake = 0.3–0.4 MAC, and is the MAC at which eyes open on verbal command during emergence from anaesthesia.
> MAC intubation = 1.3 MAC is the MAC required to prevent coughing and movement during endotracheal intubation.

Factors decreasing MAC
> Increasing age
> Pregnancy
> Hypothermia
> Hyponatraemia
> Hypothyroidism
> Hypotension
> Hypoxia
> Metabolic acidosis
> Acute alcohol intake
> Narcotics
> Ketamine
> Benzodiazepines
> α_2 agonists
> Lithium

Factors increasing MAC
> Young age (infants and children)
> Hyperthermia
> Hypernatraemia
> Chronic alcohol intake
> Increased sympathoadrenal stimulation (MAOI, acute amphetamines, ephedrine, cocaine)

Factors with no influence on MAC

> Duration of anaesthesia
> Gender
> Alkalosis
> Hypertension
> Anaemia
> Magnesium and potassium levels

What factors affect MAC?

Table 18.4   Summary of the key features of inhalational anaesthetic agents

	Halothane	Isoflurane	Enflurane	Sevoflurane	Desflurane
Chemical	Halogenated hydrocarbon	Halogenated methyl ethyl ether	Halogenated methyl ethyl ether	Polyfluorinated isopropyl methyl ether	Fluorinated methyl ethyl ether
Molecular weight	197	184	184	200	168
Boiling point (°C)	50.2	48.5	56.5	58.5	22.8
SVP at 20 °C (kP$_a$)	32.3	33.2	23.3	22.7	89.2
Oil:Gas	224	98	98	53	29
Blood:Gas	2.3	1.4	1.8	0.6	0.4
MAC in 100% O_2	0.75	1.17	1.68	1.9	6.6
MAC in 70% N_2O	0.29	0.56	0.57	0.66	2.5
% Metabolised	20	0.2	2	3–5	0.02
Toxicity	Hepatitis			Compound A	
SVR	↓	↓↓	↓↓	↓	↓ above 2.2 MAC
MAP	↓	↓	↓	↓	↓
HR	↓↓	↑↑	↑	↓	↑↑
CO	↓	↔	↔	↔	↔
Contractility	↓	↔ initially ↓ at high doses	↓	↔ initially ↓ at high doses	↔ initially ↓ (less than other agents)
Sensitise myocardium to catecholamines	Yes ++	No	Yes	No	No
Tidal volume	↓	↓	↓	↓	↓
RR	↓	↔	↑	↑	↑
Bronchodilatation	Yes	Yes	Yes	Yes	
Irritant	No	Yes	No	No	Yes++
Response to hypoxia % hypocarbia	↓	↓	↓	↓	↓
Cerebral blood flow	↑↑	↑ (>1 MAC)	↑ (>1 MAC)	↑ (>1 MAC)	↑
CMRO$_2$	↓	↓	↓	↓	↓
Epileptiform activity	No	No	Yes	No	No
Uterine tone	↓	↓	↓	↓	↓

19. NEUROMUSCULAR BLOCKING DRUGS

Describe the nicotinic acetylcholine receptor (nAChR).

The nAChR is an integral membrane protein found on the postsynaptic membrane of the neuromuscular junction. It is a ligand-gated ion channel composed of five subunits: two α, one β, one δ and one γ, which are all arranged around a central pore. Its molecular weight is about 250 000 Daltons.

When a molecule of ACh binds to each of the α subunits, the receptor undergoes conformational change, which results in opening of the central pore. This pore is a non-specific ion channel, through with Na^+, K^+ and Ca^{2+} ions can flow, causing miniature end-plate potentials. When the threshold level of depolarisation is reached, voltage-gated Na^+ channels open and the action potential is propagated across the muscle.

How does suxamethonium exert its effects?

> Suxamethonium is a depolarising neuromuscular-blocking drug. Its structure is that of two conjugated acetylcholine molecules and as such it is much more stable than the natural ligand. Suxamethonium binds to the α subunit of the nAChR and causes the ion channel to open, with resulting muscle depolarisation. This results in muscular fasciculations as the depolarisation caused by suxamethonium is not orderly.
> Suxamethonium is not broken down by acetylcholine esterase and therefore its effects at the receptor are more sustained than the natural ligand. This persistent depolarisation causes the Na^+ channels to become inactive, preventing repolarisation and rendering the neuromuscular end plate refractory to further stimulation. This produces a flaccid paralysis in the patient. With time, the drug diffuses away from the neuromuscular junction and is broken down by pseudocholinesterase (also known as plasma cholinesterase or butyrylcholinesterase) in the plasma. Now, repolarisation can occur and muscle action potentials are again possible.

What are the characteristics of the ideal neuromuscular blocker?

Physical properties:
> Cheap and easy to manufacture
> Long shelf life at room temperature
> Water soluble and therefore easy to store
> Painless on injection
> Safe if injected intra-arterially
> Ultra rapid onset time
> Predictable duration of action
> Able to reverse its effects quickly following an intubating dose
> No accumulation following infusion
> No interaction with other drugs

Biological properties:
> Analgesic
> No systemic effects other than neuromuscular blockade
> No toxic effects

How are non-depolarising neuromuscular blocking drugs classified?

They are classified into two groups according to their chemical composition:

> **Aminosteroids**, e.g. vecuronium, rocuronium, pancuronium
> **Benzylisoquinolinium esters**, e.g. atracurium, mivacurium

How do these drugs work?

> Both classes exert their effects by binding to the α subunits of the nAChR and competitively inhibiting ACh.
> The drug needs to occupy only one of the α subunits but must occupy at least 70% of all receptors, before any effect is clinically evident.
> This feature highlights the margin of safety that exists within an individual with regards to neuromuscular function. It is well demonstrated in patients with myasthenia gravis where a significant proportion of nAChR must be affected before symptoms become evident.

What factors affect the speed of onset of the drug?

Non-depolarising muscle relaxants have bulky structures and are relatively polar. Their volumes of distribution are therefore small and they are not significantly redistributed. They do not undergo first-pass metabolism, and are all administered intravenously. Hence, their speed of onset is governed by the concentration gradient between plasma and effect site.

Rocuronium is a much less potent drug than vecuronium, and therefore a higher dose of rocuronium must be given in order to achieve the same degree of muscle relaxation. At first, this sounds undesirable but this increase in intubating dose (from vecuronium 0.1 mg/kg to rocuronium 0.6 mg/kg) means that a greater number of rocuronium molecules are being given, which increases the relative concentration gradient between the plasma and the nAChR. This results in more rapid movement of rocuronium molecules onto the receptors, and therefore a faster onset of action when compared with vecuronium. At a rapid sequence intubating dose of 1 mg/kg, its speed of onset is comparable with suxamethonium.

What are ED_{50} and ED_{95}?

This is the dose of neuromuscular blocking agent required to produce either a 50% or 95% depression in twitch height when measuring train of four using a nerve stimulator (*see Study Guide 1*, Chapter 78: 'Neuromuscular blockage monitoring'). The standard intubating dose is $2 \times ED_{95}$. When high-dose rocuronium is used in order to produce intubating conditions within 60 s, a dose equivalent to $4 \times ED_{95}$ is used.

What factors affect the speed of recovery from non-depolarising muscle relaxation?

Initial dose:
The greater the dose, the longer recovery takes.

Drug metabolism:
> Aminosteroids are minimally metabolised in the liver and excreted in the bile and urine (both as unchanged and changed products). Liver and renal impairment can lead to accumulation of the drugs and therefore prolong their effects.
> Atracurium (benzylisoquinolinium ester) is broken down by Hoffman degradation, a process of spontaneous drug breakdown at body pH and temperature. Acidosis and hypothermia will slow this breakdown and prolong its effects.

Drug interactions:
> Drugs that induce liver enzymes will reduce the effects of the aminosteroids, e.g. co-administration of phenytoin results in an 80% increase in the necessary dose of aminosteroid.
> Co-administration of magnesium sulphate, which competes with calcium, will prolong the action of neuromuscular blockers by inhibiting the release of ACh from its vesicular stores at the neuromuscular junction. Only 30–50% of the normal dose of relaxant should be used.

Administration of 'reversal agents':

> Anticholinesterases: Until relatively recently the only drugs available to reverse the effects of non-depolarising neuromuscular blockers were anticholinesterases, e.g. neostigmine, which worked by increasing the concentration of ACh at the neuromuscular junction.
> Sugammadex: Licensed for use with rocuronium and vecuronium. This modified γ-cyclodextrin works by completely enveloping the aminosteroid and terminating its effects as it can no longer interact with the nAChR. The drug–drug compound is then excreted in the urine. Given 3 minutes after an intubating dose of rocuronium, it will terminate its effects in 1.5 minutes.

How does the structure of these drugs govern their effects?

> Aminosteroidal drugs are bulky and polar and therefore they do not easily cross cell membranes and their volume of distribution is low. They contain moieties that resemble ACh which interact with the nAChR.
> Atracurium has an oxygen atom in its structure that attracts neighbouring electrons, therefore destabilising the bonds between constituent atoms. This leads to breakdown of the molecule in a process known as Hoffman degradation.

Pancuronium bromide

USES
- To provide muscle relaxation to allow intubation, ventilation and surgery
- Part of the lethal injection in USA
- Long acting

ABSORPTION/ DISTRIBUTION
- Protein binding 10–40%
- V_D 0.27 L/kg

MOA
- Competitive inhibition of ACh at nicotinic receptors at NMJ
- Binds to α-subunit of receptor but does not stimulate it to open ion channel

EFFECTS
- Stimulates SNS, may block reuptake of noradrenaline
- Blocks cardiac muscarinic receptors
- Tachycardia
- Sweating, flushing
- Salivation

PANCURONIUM BROMIDE
Aminosteroid non-depolarising muscle relaxant
- Clear colourless solution: 2 mg/mL in 2 mL vials
- Store at 4°C

DOSE
- 0.1 mg/kg gives intubating conditions in 90–120 s
- Duration 100 min.

METABOLISM AND EXCRETION
- 35% hepatic metabolism to 3- and 17-hydroxy and 3,17-dihydroxypancuronium
- 3-hydroxy metabolite is half as potent as parent
- Unmetabolised drug excreted in urine
- Metabolised drug excreted in bile

CHEMICAL PROPERTIES
- Bromide salt

Suxamethonium

USES
- Rapid sequence induction for fast onset of relaxation (45 s)

MOA
- Binds to α-subunit of nicotinic receptors at neuromuscular junction, causing chaotic depolarisation of muscle, therefore fasciculation occurs before flaccid paralysis
- Not broken down by acetylcholinesterase, and more stable than endogenous ACh, so occupies receptor for longer maintaining relaxation
- Broken down by pseuodocholinesterase in plasma after diffusing away from synaptic cleft

ABSORPTION/ DISTRIBUTION
- Because of rapid hydrolysis, only 20% of dose reaches NMJ

EFFECTS
May precipitate:
- Arrhythmias by binding to muscarinic receptors – sinus and nodal bradycardia and ventricular ectopics
- Anaphylaxis
- Malignant hyperpyrexia
- Release of potassium from cells causing hyperkalaemia, especially in burn patients, effect persists from 24 hours to 2 years after injury
- Myalgia – especially in young, fit, ambulant patients
- ↑ IOP
- ↑ Intragastric pressure and LOS pressure
- Prolonged neuromuscular blockade with repeated dosing = Type 2 block, i.e. shows characteristic of non-depolarising agent, with fade on TOF. Cannot be reversed with neostigmine

SUXAMETHONIUM
(succinylcholine or scoline)
Depolarising neuromuscular blocker
- Clear colourless solution: 50 mg/mL
- Store at 4°C
- Routes: IV/IM

DOSE
- 1–2 mg/kg

METABOLISM AND EXCRETION
- Diffuses away from synaptic cleft and metabolised by plasma cholinesterases (also called pseudocholinesterase)
- Hydrolysed to choline + succinylmonocholine
- Latter metabolised further to succinic acid and choline

CHEMICAL PROPERTIES
- Made up of two acetylcholine molecules joined together by their acetyl groups
- White crystalline substance that is very soluble in water
- pH of solution = 4

Atracurium

USES
- To provide muscle relaxation to allow intubation, ventilation and surgery
- Useful in those with renal and liver disease as not reliant on these for metabolism

ABSORPTION/ DISTRIBUTION
- Protein binding 15%
- V_D 0.15 L/kg

MOA
- Competitive inhibition of ACh at nicotinic receptors at NMJ
- Binds to α-subunits of receptor but does not stimulate it to open ion channel

EFFECTS
- Causes histamine release, can precipitate hypotension and bronchospasm in susceptible individuals. Some avoid its use in asthmatics. Slow IV injection minimises histamine release.
- Associated with critical illness myopathy.

METABOLISM AND EXCRETION
- Two modes of metabolism:
- Ester hydrolysis (60% of dose) in plasma by non-specific esterases to laudanosine, a quaternary acid and alcohol.
- Hofmann degradation, i.e. spontaneous breakdown to laudanosine and monoacrylate. This occurs at body temp and pH. Acidosis and cold slow the rate of degradation.
- Laudanosine can cause seizures, but not at clinical levels.

ATRACURIUM
Benzylisoquinolinium non-depolarising muscle relaxant
- Clear colourless solution 10 mg/mL in 2.5, 5 and 25 mL vials.
- Store at 4°C to avoid Hofmann degradation.

DOSE
- 0.5 mg/kg provides intubating conditions in 90–120 s.

CHEMICAL PROPERTIES
- 4 chiral centres and so 10 stereoisomers make up the solution
- Cis atracurium is available. This single isomer was developed to avoid unwanted histamine release and its side effects.

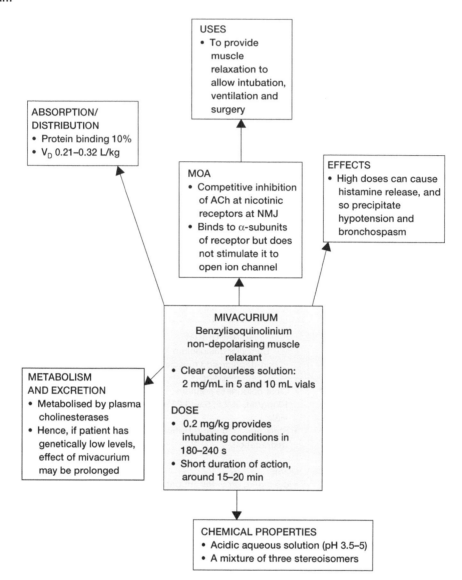

USES
- To provide muscle relaxation to allow intubation, ventilation and surgery

ABSORPTION/ DISTRIBUTION
- Protein binding 10%
- V_D 0.21–0.32 L/kg

MOA
- Competitive inhibition of ACh at nicotinic receptors at NMJ
- Binds to α-subunits of receptor but does not stimulate it to open ion channel

EFFECTS
- High doses can cause histamine release, and so precipitate hypotension and bronchospasm

MIVACURIUM
Benzylisoquinolinium non-depolarising muscle relaxant
- Clear colourless solution: 2 mg/mL in 5 and 10 mL vials

DOSE
- 0.2 mg/kg provides intubating conditions in 180–240 s
- Short duration of action, around 15–20 min

METABOLISM AND EXCRETION
- Metabolised by plasma cholinesterases
- Hence, if patient has genetically low levels, effect of mivacurium may be prolonged

CHEMICAL PROPERTIES
- Acidic aqueous solution (pH 3.5–5)
- A mixture of three stereoisomers

Vecuronium bromide

ABSORPTION/
DISTRIBUTION
• Protein binding
  10%
• V_D 0.23 L/kg

USES
• To provide muscle
  relaxation to allow
  intubation, ventilation
  and surgery

MOA
• Competitive inhibition
  of ACh at nicotinic
  receptors at NMJ
• Binds to α-subunit of
  receptor but does not
  stimulate it to open
  ion channel

EFFECTS
• Critical illness
  myopathy if given for a
  prolonged period

VECURONIUM BROMIDE
Aminosteroid
non-depolarising muscle
relaxant
• White powder: 10 mg/vial,
  for reconstitution with
  water

DOSE
• 0.1 mg/kg allows
  intubation in 90–120 s
• Duration 45 min

METABOLISM
AND EXCRETION
• Hepatic metabolism by
  deacetylation to
  3 and 17-hydroxy and
  3,17-hydroxyvecuronium
• Clinically insignificant
  metabolites
• Excreted in bile (70%)
  and urine (30%)

CHEMICAL PROPERTIES
• Monoquaternary analogue of pancuronium
  – differs by one methyl group

Rocuronium bromide

ABSORPTION/
DISTRIBUTION
• Protein binding
  10%
• V_D 0.2 L/kg

USES
• To provide muscle
  relaxation to allow
  intubation, ventilation
  and surgery

MOA
• Competitive inhibition
  of ACh at nicotinic
  receptors at NMJ
• Binds to α-subunit of
  receptor but does not
  stimulate it to open ion
  channel

EFFECTS
• At high doses can
  exert vagolytic effect,
  causing tachycardia
• Otherwise, no
  systemic effects

ROCURONIUM BROMIDE
Aminosteroid
non-depolarising muscle
relaxant
• Clear, colourless solution:
  10 mg/mL
• Stored at 4°C

DOSE
• 0.6 mg/kg allows
  intubation in 90–120 s
• 0.9–1.2 mg/kg in 60 s
  Duration 45 min

METABOLISM
AND EXCRETION
• Only 5% metabolised
  by liver
• Excreted in bile (60%)
  and urine (40%)
• Duration of action may
  be increased in
  liver/renal failure

CHEMICAL PROPERTIES
• Monoquaternary amine analogue of vecuronium
• 7x less potent than vecuronium, so a higher dose needs
  to be given to achieve relaxation. The higher number of
  molecules given causes an increased concentration
  gradient between blood and NMJ and so results in a
  faster onset of action by rules of kinetics.

20. CHOLINESTERASE INHIBITORS (ANTICHOLINESTERASES) AND REVERSAL AGENTS

How do anticholinesterases exert their effects?

> They inhibit the action of acetylcholinesterase by occupying its active site, which prevents it from breaking down acetylcholine (ACh).
> These agents are used to reverse the effects of non-depolarising neuromuscular blocking drugs, as they increase the amount of ACh available to compete with the muscle relaxant at neuromuscular junction.
> They are also used in the diagnosis and treatment of myasthenia gravis and form an active ingredient in pesticides and nerve gases.

How are these drugs classified?

Anticholinesterases are classified according to their duration of action:

Short acting:
> Edrophonium (trade name Tensilon)
  • Duration: 10–20 minutes.
  • Mode of action: Competitive antagonist of ACh at the active site of acetylcholinesterase.
  • Uses: In the diagnosis of myasthenia gravis (Tensilon test) – following administration, muscle power improves.

Medium acting:
> Neostigmine
  • Duration: 1–2 hours.
  • Mode of action: Carbamlyates the active site of the enzyme. Once bonded, it is hydrolysed like ACh, but the process takes much longer. It also inhibits the action of plasma pseudocholinesterase and so will prolong the effects of suxamethonium and mivacurium.
  • Uses: Reversal of competitive neuromuscular blocking drugs and treatment of constipation on the ICU.
> Pyridostigmine
  • Duration: 2–3 hours.
  • Mode of action: As for neostigmine.
  • Uses: Orally, in the treatment of myasthenia gravis.

> Physostigmine
  • Duration: 0.5–5 hours.
  • Mode of action: As for neostigmine.
  • Uses: Topical eye drops in the treatment of glaucoma.

Long acting:
> Echothiophate
  • Duration: Weeks.
  • Mode of action: Phosphorylation of the active site of the enzyme. The bond is covalent and the enzyme takes weeks to hydrolyse the drug.
  • Uses: Treatment of glaucoma.

This class also includes:
> Sarin, VX – nerve gases used in chemical warfare.
> Tetraethyl pyrophosphate (TEPP) – an insecticide.

In toxic doses (e.g. organophosphorus poisoning), anticholinesterases can cause SLUDGE syndrome (salivation, lacrimation, urination, defecation, gastrointestinal upset, emesis) and cause death by paralysis of the respiratory muscles. Treatment is with antimuscarinic agents, such as atropine and pralidoxime.

What are the side effects of a conventional dose of neostigmine?

Cardiovascular:
> Bradycardia
> Hypotension

Respiratory:
> Bronchoconstriction
> Increased secretions

Neurological:
> Miosis and blurred vision
> Low dose: muscle contraction
> High dose: large amounts of ACh at NMJ may render neuromuscular transmission obsolete.

Gastrointestinal:
> Increased secretions
> Peristalsis
> Nausea and vomiting

Other:
> Sweating

To offset these unpleasant effects, neostigmine is usually given with an antimuscarinic agent such as glycopyrrolate.

Neostigmine

USES
- Reversal of neuromuscular blockade caused by non-depolarising muscle relaxants
- Myasthenia gravis
- Paralytic ileus

MOA
- Binds to esteratic site of acetylcholinesterase (AChE), the enzyme which breaks down acetylcholine (ACh)
- Neostigmine is hydrolysed by AChE, but much more slowly than ACh would be
- As enzymes' active sites are occupied by neostigmine, more ACh is available at the neuromuscular junction (NMJ)
- Increased quantity of ACh at NMJ allows more efficient competition with non-depolarising muscle relaxants

ABSORPTION/ DISTRIBUTION
- Poorly absorbed orally
- Oral bioavailability 1–2%
- Protein binding 10%
- V_D 0.4–1 L/kg
- Max effect in 7–11 min, lasts 4 hours
- $t_{1/2}$ 15–80 min

EFFECTS
CVS
- Bradycardia
- Hypotension
RS
- Bronchoconstriction
- Increased secretions
CNS
- Miosis and blurred vision
- Low dose: muscle contraction
- High dose: large amounts of ACh at NMJ may block neuromuscular transmission as receptors flooded
GI
- Increased secretions
- Peristalsis
- Nausea and vomiting
OTHER
- Sweating

METABOLISM AND EXCRETION
- Metabolised by plasma esterases
- Small amount of hepatic metabolism, these products excreted in bile
- Remainder excreted in urine

NEOSTIGMINE
Anticholinesterase quaternary amine
- Tablets: 15 mg
- Solution: 2.5 mg/mL
- Mixed with glycopyrrolate: 2.5 mg neostigmine + 0.5 mg glycopyrrolate/mL

DOSE
- 0.05 mg/kg IV

CHEMICAL PROPERTIES
- Nil

Edrophonium

USES
- Reversal of neuromuscular blockade caused by non-depolarising muscle relaxants
- Diagnosis of myasthenia gravis ('Tensilon test' – following drug administration, muscle strength improves. Tested by EMG)
- Differentiating between myasthenic crises (where strength improves) and cholinergic crisis in patients with myasthenia gravis (where it worsens)

EFFECTS
Mainly result from $\uparrow$ activation of muscarinic receptors by ACh
CVS
- Bradycardia
- Hypotension
- Cardiac arrest reported
RS
- Bronchoconstriction
- Increased secretions
CNS
- Miosis and blurred vision
- Low dose: muscle contraction
- High dose: large amounts of ACh at NMJ may render neuromuscular transmission obsolete
GI
- Increased secretions
- Peristalsis
- Nausea and vomiting
OTHER
- Sweating

ABSORPTION/ DISTRIBUTION
- V_D 0.9–1.3 L/kg
- Max effect in 2 min, lasts 10 min
- $t_{1/2}$ 110 min

MOA
- Binds reversibly to esteratic site of acetylcholinesterase, (AChE), the enzyme which breaks down acetylcholine (ACh)
- Competes with ACh for this binding site hence reducing rate of breakdown of ACh
- So, more ACh available to activate nACh receptor and cause muscle contraction

EDROPHONIUM
Anticholinesterase-quaternary amine
- Solution: 10 mg/mL

DOSE
- Tensilon test = 2 mg followed by 8 mg if no improvement in strength

METABOLISM AND EXCRETION
- No information

CHEMICAL PROPERTIES
- Nil

Sugammadex

USES
- Reversal of neuromuscular blockade caused by rocuronium and vecuronium
- Can be used confidently to reverse effects, even following an intubating dose of rocuronium

EFFECTS
CVS
- Cardiovascularly stable
- Avoids need to give anticholinesterase and antimuscarinic to reverse neuromuscular blockade, with their attendant side-effects

OTHER
- Also has affinity for pancuronium, though not licensed for its reversal
- Affinity: rocuronium>vecuronium>pancuronium
- Produces rapid reversal because encapsulating the muscle relaxant in the plasma creates a concentration gradient between plasma and NMJ, which causes rocuronium/vecuronium to diffuse away from NMJ into plasma

MOA
- Its ring-like structure enables drug to encapsulate rocuronium and vecuronium in its lipophilic core
- The active site of the muscle relaxant is bound to carboxyl groups in the cyclodextrin so it cannot interact with the acetylcholine receptors at the neuromuscular junction (NMJ)
- Causes reversal of neuromuscular blockade

ABSORPTION/ DISTRIBUTION
- Biologically inactive
- No protein binding
- $t_{1/2}$ 1.8 hours

METABOLISM AND EXCRETION
- Both cyclodextrin and cyclodextrin-aminosteroid complex excreted in urine

SUGAMMADEX
Modified γ-cyclodextrin
Trade name: Bridion
- Approved for use in Europe in July 2008
- Clear colourless solution: 100 mg/mL in 2 mL or 5 mL vials

DOSE
- Moderate block: 2 twitches, 2 mg/kg
- Deep block: 1–2 post-tetanic count, 4 mg/kg
- Immediate reversal from RSI, 16 mg/kg
- At these doses recurrence of blockade is not a clinical problem

CHEMICAL PROPERTIES
- Nil

21. ANTIMUSCARINIC DRUGS

To answer a question on this subject well, you need to know the structure and function of the autonomic nervous system (ANS). This is covered in a separate chapter (see Study Guide 1, Chapter 35). This question could easily go on to explore other drugs that modulate the ANS, such as:

> Nicotinic AChR antagonists acting at ganglia, e.g. trimetaphan
> mAChR agonists, e.g. pilocarpine
> Adrenoceptor antagonists, e.g. α and β-blockers
> Adrenoceptor agonists, e.g. adrenaline.

How do antimuscarinic drugs work?

> Antimuscarinic agents are competitive antagonists of acetylcholine (ACh) at muscarinic acetylcholine receptors (mAChR). These are located in post-ganglionic target tissues innervated by the parasympathetic nervous system (PNS) and also in the sympathetically innervated sweat glands.
> These drugs are also called 'parasympatholytic' agents because they reduce the activity of the PNS.

What are the clinical uses of these agents?

Antimuscarinic agents have both anaesthetic and non-anaesthetic uses:

> **Premedication**, e.g. hyoscine
  • Used to produce sedation and amnesia.
  • Hyoscine comes in two formulations: hyoscine hydrobromide, which crosses the blood–brain barrier (BBB) to produce central effects such as sedation, amnesia and anti-emesis; and hyoscine butylbromide (Buscopan®), which does not cross the BBB.
> **Bradycardia treatment**, e.g. atropine
> **Anti-sialogogue**, e.g. glycopyrrolate.
  • Used prophylactically to reduce excessive secretions in procedures such as fibre-optic intubation.
  • Hyoscine is used in palliative care to reduce excessive secretions (death rattle).
> **Bronchodilator**, e.g. ipratropium bromide.
> **Antiemetic**, e.g. hyoscine
  • Used to treat motion sickness, post-operative nausea and vomiting, and opioid-induced nausea.
> **Anti-spasmodic**, e.g. hyoscine
  • Used to treat colicky abdominal pain.
  • Used to fascilitate upper gastrointestinal endoscopy.
> **Co-administered with anticholinesterases**, e.g. glycopyrrolate with neostigmine
  • Used to attenuate the muscarinic effects of neostigmine.
> **Anti-parkinsonian drug**, e.g. benztropine, procyclidine and benzhexol.
> **Mydriatic**, e.g. tropicamide.
> **Antidote to organophosphorus and nerve gas poisoning**
  • Troops at risk of chemical warfare carry mini-jets of atropine and obidoxime that can be injected into the thigh.

Can you describe the structure of hyoscine, atropine and glycopyrrolate?

> Atropine and hyoscine (also known as scopolamine) are naturally occurring tertiary amines extracted from plants of the deadly nightshade family. They are formed from the esters of tropic acid and tropine or scopine respectively. Being tertiary amines, these agents are able to cross the BBB and can produce central anticholinergic effects.
> Glycopyrrolate is a synthetic quaternary amine that cannot readily cross the BBB and so central anticholinergic effects are negligible with this agent.

Compare and contrast hyoscine, atropine and glycopyrrolate.

Table 21.1 The properties of hyoscine, atropine and glycopyrrolate compared

Property	Hyoscine	Atropine	Glycopyrrolate
Structure	3° amine	3° amine	4° amine
Formulation	Hyoscine hydrobromide (crosses BBB) Hyoscine butylbromide (does not cross BBB)	Atropine sulphate	Glycopyrrolate bromide
Route	PO, IM, IV, TD	PO, IM, IV	IM, IV
Adult IV dose (µg/kg)	5–10	5–20	3–10
Bioavailability	10%	10–25%	5%
% protein binding	11%	50%	Not available
V_D (L/kg)	2	2–4	0.2–0.6
Cl (L/kg)	45	70	0.9
$T_{1/2}$ (h)	2.5	2.5	1
Sedation/Amnesia	+++	+	0
Anti-emesis	++	+	0
Anticholinergic syndrome	++	++	0
Mydriasis	+++	+	0
Antisialagogue	+++	+	++
Bronchodilation	+	++	++
Tachycardia	+	+++	++
Placental transfer	++	++	0
Metabolism	+++ Liver esterases	+++ Liver esterases	Minimal
Excretion	Urine (tiny fraction unchanged)	Urine (tiny fraction unchanged)	Urine and bile (majority unchanged)

What are the major side effects of these agents?

The major side effects produced by these agents result from their antagonistic action on the 'rest and digest' activity of glands, smooth muscle and cardiac muscle. Therefore, their side effect profile can be worked out logically and classified systematically:

> **Neurological:**
>   • 3° amines can cross the BBB and produce an acute central anti-cholinergic syndrome. The central features of this syndrome include altered mental status, disorientation, hallucinations, agitation, ataxia, somnolence and coma. The peripheral features of this syndrome include dry mouth, mydriasis, blurred vision, paralytic ileus, urinary retention, tachycardia, and hot, dry and vasodilated skin.
> **Eye:**
>   • Mydriasis causing photophobia and loss of accommodation (cycloplegia) resulting in blurred vision and diplopia
>   • Dry eyes (xerophthalmia) due to reduced lacrimal secretion
>   • Risk of raised intra-ocular pressure in patients with closed angle glaucoma
> **Respiratory:**
>   • Increased anatomical dead space
> **Cardiovascular:**
>   • Tachycardia
> **Gastrointestinal:**
>   • Decreased bowel movement
>   • Paralytic ileus
>   • Reduced lower oesophageal sphincter pressure – risk of exacerbating reflux in susceptible individuals.
> **Genito-urinary:**
>   • Reduced urinary tract peristalsis and detrusor muscle tone combined with increased sphincter tone to cause urinary retention.
> **Skin:**
>   • Impaired sweating results in hot, dry and vasodilated skin.
>   • Pyrexia may follow especially in children or in cases of overdose.

Atropine

ABSORPTION/ DISTRIBUTION
- Well absorbed orally
- Oral bioavailability 10–25%
- Protein binding 50%
- V_D 2–4 L/kg

USES
- Premed to decrease secretions
- Treatment of bradycardia
- In ALS algorithm (PEA/asystole)
- Treatment of organophosphate poisoning

EFFECTS
CVS
- Tachycardia
- Effect last 2–3 hours
- May precipitate arrhythmias by decreasing AV conduction time

RS
- Bronchodilation
- ↑RR

CNS
- Crosses BBB causing central anticholinergic syndrome
- Antiemetic
- Antiparkinsonian effects

GI
- Antisialagogue
- ↓Tone lower oesophageal sphincter

METABOLIC
- Inhibits sweating may cause hyperpyrexia in children

ANTIMUSCARINIC
- Dry mouth
- Urinary retention
- Blurred vision

MOA
- Competitive antagonist at muscarinic receptors ('vagolytic')

METABOLISM AND EXCRETION
- Hepatic metabolism
- Metabolised and unchanged drug excreted in urine

ATROPINE
Synthetic tertiary amine
- Solution: 0.6 mg/mL
- Tablets: 600 µg

DOSE
- 0.2–0.6 mg IV or IM (adult)
- 20 µg/kg (children)

CHEMICAL PROPERTIES
- Racemic mixture of D and L atropine
- Only L is active

Glycopyrrolate

USES
- Premed to decrease oral secretions
- To attenuate effects of anticholinesterases, i.e. when given to reverse non-depolarising muscle relaxants
- Bradycardia
- Hyperhydrosis

EFFECTS
CVS
- Tachycardia
- Effect lasts 2–3 hours
RS
- Bronchodilation
CNS
- Doesn't cross BBB but still causes headache and sedation
GI
- Antisialagogue
METABOLIC
- Inhibits sweating
ANTIMUSCARINIC
- Dry mouth
- Urinary retention
- Blurred vision

ABSORPTION/ DISTRIBUTION
- Poor oral absorption
- Oral bioavailability 5%

MOA
- Competitive antagonist at muscarinic receptors ('vagolytic')
- Does not cross BBB

GLYCOPYRROLATE
Synthetic quaternary amine
- Solution: 0.2 mg/mL
- Mixed with neostigmine: 0.5 mg glyco + 250 mg neo/mL

DOSE
- 0.2–0.4 mg IV or IM (adult)
- 4–10 µg/kg (children)

METABOLISM AND EXCRETION
- Minimal metabolism
- Excreted unchanged in urine

CHEMICAL PROPERTIES
- Nil

22. OPIOIDS

What is the difference between an opiate and an opioid?	The term **opiate** refers to naturally occurring compounds that are derivatives of opium, which have morphine-like properties. Opium comes from the sap of the opium poppy, and examples of opiates are morphine and codeine. An **opioid** is a synthetic substance that stimulates the opioid receptor, e.g. fentanyl and alfentanil.
How do opioids exert their effects?	Opioids work by stimulating presynaptic G_i-protein-coupled opioid receptors. Binding of the ligand causes the following events: > Closure of voltage-gated Ca^{2+} channels > Decreased cAMP production > Stimulation of K^+ efflux from the cell > Hyperpolarisation of the cell membrane. > This leads to decreased excitability of the cell and therefore decreased neurotransmitter release and pain transmission.
Classify the opioid receptors.	There are four main types of opioid receptor, and some of these have subtypes. The receptors were named for the process through which they were discovered: > **µ receptor** (subtypes μ_1, μ_2, μ_3): morphine was used to identify it > **κ receptor** (subtypes κ_1, κ_2, κ_3): ketocyclazocine was used to identify it > **δ receptor** (subtypes δ_1, δ_2): found in the vas **d**eferens of mice > **NOP receptor**: nociceptin orphanin FQ peptide receptor (most recently identified). The accepted nomenclature for these receptors is now **MOP** (µ), **KOP** (κ), **DOP** (δ) and **NOP** (N/OFQ), as decided by the International Union of Pharmacology (*see* Table 22.1).
What are the unwanted effects of opioids?	Refer to the spider diagram for morphine (p. 81) for a list of side effects.
What is tolerance?	Tolerance refers to a decreasing response to repeated dosing of a drug. Over time, a larger dose is needed to produce the same effect. There are two theories as to how this develops: either because of receptor down-regulation or because with repeated doses of opioid there is uncoupling of the receptor from its G protein. Morphine seems to cause uncoupling, but not down-regulation of its receptors.

Table 22.1 Opioid receptor classification

Receptor type	Location	Action when stimulated
MOP	Brain – especially areas involved with sensory and motor perception and integration. Abundant in periaqueductal grey. Spinal cord	μ_1 > Analgesia > Physical dependence μ_2 > Respiratory depression > Reduced peristalsis > Euphoria > Meiosis
DOP	Brain	> Analgesia > Antidepressant > Physical dependence
KOP	Brain Spinal cord	> Spinal analgesia > Sedation > Meiosis
NOP	Brain Spinal cord	> Anxiety > Depression > Affects learning and memory > Involved in tolerance > Natural ligand may set body's pain threshold, and so administration of an agonist may mean less MOP agonism is needed to achieve pain relief.

What is dependence?

A physically dependent patient will need to repeatedly administer the drug to avoid suffering from withdrawal symptoms.

What is addiction?

Addiction is characterised by the patient's behaviour resulting from their dependence. An addict will:

> Crave and seek out the drug
> Have no control over their drug use
> Use the drug compulsively
> Continue to use the drug even if it is causing them harm.

What are the symptoms of opioid withdrawal?

Symptoms include:

> Anxiety and fear
> Adrenergic hyperactivity
> Malaise
> Abdominal cramps
> Sweating
> Yawning

How will you manage post-operative pain control in an opioid-dependent patient?

When treating dependent patients, their baseline pre-existing opioid dosage should be continued and additional pain relief should be administered as required. The patient will be tolerant to opioids and so may need more than the 'average patient' to achieve pain relief. For this reason pethidine should be avoided as large doses may cause the proconvulsant metabolite nor-pethidine to accumulate. It is sensible to include simple analgesia and regional techniques where possible.

If the patient is on a methadone programme, ascertain their daily requirements and continue this dosage perioperatively. If the patient is abstinent, they may be reluctant to use opioids for pain relief, but there is no evidence to suggest that the appropriate use of opioids will precipitate a relapse.

Morphine

USES
- Analgesia
- Sedation on ITU
- Palliative care
- CCF

ABSORPTION/DISTRIBUTION
- Well absorbed orally (from small bowel as ionised in stomach)
- Extensive first-pass metabolism
- Oral bioavailability at 15–20%
- 20–40%PPB
- V_D 3.4–4.7 L/kg
- Low lipid solubility
- Peak effect 10–30 min, duration 3–4 hours

MOA
- Agonist at MOP and KOP G-protein coupled opioid receptors
- Binding of the ligand causes the following events:
- Closure of voltage-gated Ca^{2+} channels
- Decreased cAMP production
- Stimulation of K^+ efflux from the cell
- Hyperpolarisation of the cell membrane and decreased excitability of cell decreasing neurotransmitter release and pain transmission

EFFECTS
CVS
- No direct effects
- If histamine release occurs, may cause hypotension
- Mild bradycardia secondary to $\downarrow$ sympathetic tone

RS
- Dose dependent respiratory depression ($\downarrow$ RR > $\downarrow$ VT)
- $\downarrow$ Sensitivity to pCO_2
- Antitussive
- Bronchospasm with histamine release

CNS
- Analgesia
- Sedation
- Euphoria
- Hallucinations
- Meiosis: Edinger-Westphal nucleus
- Seizures and muscular rigidity with high dose

GI
- $\downarrow$ Motility
- $\downarrow$ Gastric acid, pancreatic and bile secretion
- Nausea and vomiting: CTZ stimulation via $5-HT_3$ and dopamine receptors

GU
- $\uparrow$ Tone in uterus, bladder detrusor and sphincter muscles – can cause retention

SKIN
- Pruritis
- Rash

ENDO
- $\downarrow$ ACTH
- $\downarrow$ Gonadotrophic hormones
- $\uparrow$ ADH causing hypernatraemia and water secretion

METABOLISM AND EXCRETION
- Hepatic metabolism to:
  - morphine-3-glucuronide (inactive) and
  - morphine-6-glucuronide (active with 13x potency of morphine)
- Excreted in urine
- Neonates have $\uparrow$ sensitivity, because of immature hepatic metabolism
- Dose with care in liver impairment

MORPHINE
Naturally occurring opiate
- Tablets: 5/10/30/60/200 mg
- Syrup: 2/10/20 mg/mL
- Suppository: 15/30 mg
- Solution: 10/15/30 mg/mL for IV and neuro-axial use NB preservative free for neuro-axial use

DOSE
- Oral: 5–40 mg/4 hourly
- Rectal: 15–30 mg/4 hourly
- IV: 0.05–0.1 mg/kg/4 hourly
- IM/SC: 0.1–0.2 mg/kg/4 hourly
- Intrathecal 0.1–1 mg
- Epidural 1–5 mg

CHEMICAL PROPERTIES
- Naturally occurring phenanthrene derivative
- Weak base, pK_a 8.0 $\therefore$ ionised in stomach

Diamorphine

ABSORPTION/ DISTRIBUTION
- Well absorbed
- Extensive first-pass metabolism
- Bioavailability low
- Protein binding 40%
- $t_{\frac{1}{2}}$ 3 min

USES
- Analgesia
- Sedation on ITU
- Palliative care
- CCF
- Drug of abuse as causes euphoria

MOA
- Metabolites act at MOP or KOP receptors
- Diamorphine itself has no affinity for opioid receptors

EFFECTS
- As for morphine
- Thought to cause less nausea and vomiting and constipation than morphine

METABOLISM AND EXCRETION
- Hydrolysed by plasma enzymes and by RBCs, (probably by esterases and pseudocholinesterases) to 6-O-acetylmorphine, the active form of the drug
- 6-O-acetylmorphine glucuronidated to morphine
- 50–60% excreted in urine as morphine derivative

DIAMORPHINE
- Tablets: 10 mg
- Powder: 5/10/30/100/500 mg vials

DOSE
- 2.5–5 mg IV for pulmonary oedema/MI
- 0.1–0.4 mg intrathecally
- 1–3 mg epidurally
- Can give SC as very lipid-soluble

CHEMICAL PROPERTIES
- Synthetic diacetylated morphine derivative
- Prodrug

Alfentanil

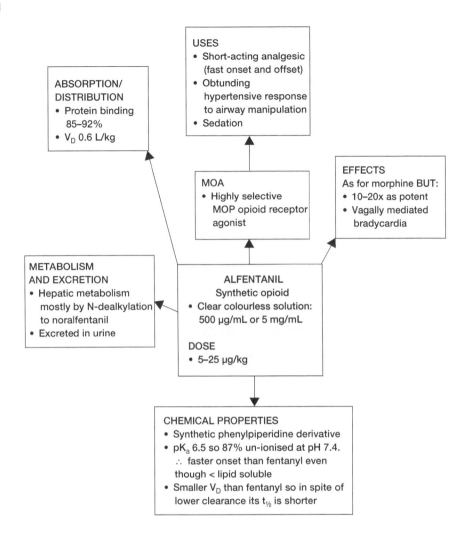

ABSORPTION/
DISTRIBUTION
• Protein binding
  85–92%
• V_D 0.6 L/kg

USES
• Short-acting analgesic
  (fast onset and offset)
• Obtunding
  hypertensive response
  to airway manipulation
• Sedation

MOA
• Highly selective
  MOP opioid receptor
  agonist

EFFECTS
As for morphine BUT:
• 10–20x as potent
• Vagally mediated
  bradycardia

METABOLISM
AND EXCRETION
• Hepatic metabolism
  mostly by N-dealkylation
  to noralfentanil
• Excreted in urine

ALFENTANIL
Synthetic opioid
• Clear colourless solution:
  500 µg/mL or 5 mg/mL

DOSE
• 5–25 µg/kg

CHEMICAL PROPERTIES
• Synthetic phenylpiperidine derivative
• pK_a 6.5 so 87% un-ionised at pH 7.4.
  ∴ faster onset than fentanyl even
  though < lipid soluble
• Smaller V_D than fentanyl so in spite of
  lower clearance its $t_{1/2}$ is shorter

Fentanyl

ABSORPTION/
DISTRIBUTION
- Absorbed orally, from small intestine
- Bioavailability 33%
- Protein binding 80–95%
- V_D 0.88–4.41 L/kg
- Short duration of action due to redistribution

USES
- Perioperative analgesia
- Obtunds hypertensive response to airway manipulation
- Opioid-based anaesthesia
- Sedation by infusion
- Chronic pain

EFFECTS
As for morphine BUT:
- 50–80x as potent
- Less histamine release
- Decreases stress response to surgery
- Associated with bradycardia
- Chest wall rigidity with high doses

MOA
- Potent agonist at MOP receptor

METABOLISM
AND EXCRETION
- Hepatic metabolism
- N-dealkylation to norfentanyl (inactive) then hydroxylation and amide hydrolysis to hydroxypropionyl derivatives
- Inactive metabolites excreted in urine

FENTANYL
Synthetic opioid
- Clear colourless solution: 50 µg/mL
- Patches: 25/50/75/100 µg/hr lasting 72 hours
- Lozenges/lollypops: 200 µg–1.6 mg over 15 min
- Patient-controlled transdermal system (PCTS): 40 µg over 10 min

DOSE
- As adjunct during induction of anaesthesia 1–100 µg/kg
- Pain relief, 1 µg/kg, repeat dose titrating to pain
- Spinal 10–30 µg
- Epidural 25–100 µg

CHEMICAL PROPERTIES
- Synthetic phenylpiperidine
- Highly lipid soluble (600x morphine)
- Highly ionised in stomach (99.9%)
- pK_a 8.4 (9% un-ionised at pH 7.4)

Remifentanil

ABSORPTION/
DISTRIBUTION
- Only given IV
- $t_{\frac{1}{2}}$ 2 hours
- Effects last only
  10 min from
  termination of infusion
- Context insensitive
  half-life

USES
- Analgesia during general
  anaesthesia
- Hypotensive anaesthesia
- Sedation on ICU and for
  procedures, e.g. awake
  fibre optic intubation

EFFECTS
As for morphine BUT:
- 50–80x as potent
- Bradycardia (may be
  profound) especially
  following bolus

MOA
- Pure MOP opioid
  receptor agonist

REMIFENTANIL
Synthetic opioid
- White crystalline powder:
  1/2/5 mg per vial,
  reconstitute with
  0.9% saline
- Give as IV infusion

DOSE
- 0.05–2 µg/kg/min

METABOLISM
AND EXCRETION
- Undergoes rapid ester
  hydrolysis by non-specific
  plasma/tissue esterases
  to carboxylic acid
  derivatives. These are
  plentiful and ∴ not
  saturated by infusion
- Excreted in urine

CHEMICAL PROPERTIES
- Because of rapid hydrolysis, effect of infusion is
  gone within 10 min of discontinuation. There is no
  residual analgesia

Pethidine

ABSORPTION/ DISTRIBUTION
- Oral bioavailability 50% (subject to first-pass metabolism)
- Protein binding 50–70%
- V_D 4 L/kg
- $t_{1/2}$ 2.4–7 hours
- Crosses placenta where norpethidine accumulates in fetus. Fetal levels peak 4 hourly after maternal dosing. Fetal $t_{1/2}$ 3x that of mother

USES
- Analgesia especially in labour
- Antispasmodic in renal and biliary colic
- Treatment of post-operative shivering

MOA
- Agonist at MOP and KOP opioid receptors
- NB not reversed by naloxone

EFFECTS
CVS
- Orthostatic hypotension
- Tachycardia secondary to anticholinergic effects

RS
- Respiratory depression
- $\downarrow V_T > \downarrow$ RR
- $\downarrow$ Response to pCO_2 and pO_2

CNS
- 1/10th potency of morphine
- More euphoria
- Less nausea and vomiting
- Miosis and corneal anaesthesia

GI
- Gastric stasis
- Less constipating than morphine

GU
- $\downarrow$ Ureteric tone
- $\uparrow$ Amplitude of contractions of pregnancy

OTHER
- $\uparrow$ ADH
- $\downarrow$ Steroid synthesis
- Severe hypertension with MAOIs
- Norpethide is proconvulsant ∴ caution in high doses

PETHIDINE
Synthetic phenylpiperidine derivative
- Tablets: 50 mg
- Solution: 10/50 mg/mL

DOSE
Adult:
- Oral: 50–150 mg 4 hourly
- IM: 25–150 mg 4 hourly
- IV: 25–100 mg 4 hourly
- Epidural: 25 mg

Child:
- Oral: 0.5–2 mg/kg
- IM: 0.5–2 mg/kg

METABOLISM AND EXCRETION
- Hepatic metabolism by N-demethylation to norpethidine (50% as potent as parent) then hydrolysed to pethidinic acid
- Excreted in urine, accumulates in renal failure

CHEMICAL PROPERTIES
- Nil

Codeine

USES
- Analgesia
- Antitussive
- Treatment of diarrhoea/high output stomas

ABSORPTION/ DISTRIBUTION
- Well absorbed
- Oral bioavailability 60–70%
- 7%PPB
- V_D 5.4 L/kg

EFFECTS
CVS
- IV can cause profound hypotension secondary to histamine release ∴ not used via this route

RS
- Antitussive
- Mild depression
- ↓ Response to ↑ pCO_2/↓ pO_2

CNS
- 10x less potent than morphine
- Dizziness

GI
- Constipation
- Nausea and vomiting

MISCELLANEOUS
- Withdrawn from use in children under 12 years old, children with sleep apnoea under 18 years old and breast feeding mothers because of unpredictable metabolism and potentially fatal risk of respiratory depression.

MOA
- Codeine has low affinity for opioid receptors
- 10% metabolised to morphine – acts via MOP and KOP opioid receptors
- Antitussive effects via specific codeine receptors

METABOLISM AND EXCRETION
- Hepatic metabolism in three ways:
  1. 10–20% glucuronidation to codeine-6-glucuronide
  2. 10–20% N-demethylation to norcodeine
  3. 5–15% O-demethylation to MORPHINE
- NB genetic variability with P450 enzyme CYPZD6 means resulting dose of morphine is variable. 9% UK population and 30% of Chinese are slow metabolisers so codeine will not provide effective analgesia

CODEINE
- Tablets: 15/30/60 mg
- Syrup: 5 mg/mL
- Solution for injection: 60 mg/mL
- Preparations + paracetamol/ibuprofen/aspirin

DOSE
- 30–60 mg 6 hourly (adults)
- 1 mg/kg 6 hourly (children over 12 years old)

CHEMICAL PROPERTIES
- Naturally occurring phenanthene alkaloid – a methylated morphine derivative

Tramadol

USES
• Analgesia

ABSORPTION/
DISTRIBUTION
• Oral bioavailability
70–90%
• V_D 4 L/kg
• t_½ 5–6 hours

MOA
• Weak agonist at all opiate
receptors, increased affinity
for MOP
• Inhibits reuptake of
noradrenaline and 5-HT
• Stimulates presynaptic
release of 5-HT, so
modulates pain via
descending
inhibitory pathways

EFFECTS
As for morphine BUT:
• 1/10th potency of
morphine
• Less respiratory
depression
• Less constipation
• Lowers seizure
threshold, so relatively
contraindicated in
epileptics parents

METABOLISM
AND EXCRETION
• Hepatic metabolism
• 1 active metabolite –
O-desmethyltramadol
• Excreted in urine (90%)
and faeces (10%)

TRAMADOL
Synthetic opioid

• Tablets: 50/100 mg,
standard and modified
release
• Solution: 100 mg/2 mL

DOSE
• 50–100 mg 6 hourly

CHEMICAL PROPERTIES
• A synthetic opioid cyclohexanol
• Racemic mixture

Naloxone

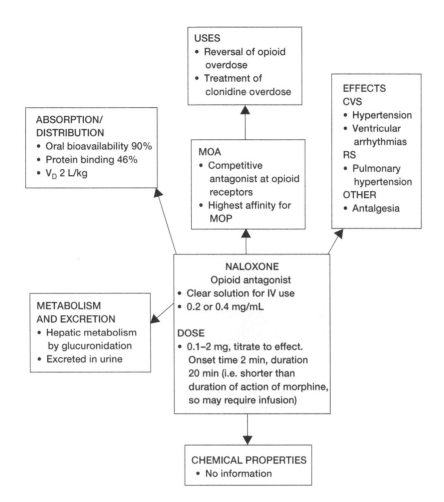

USES
- Reversal of opioid overdose
- Treatment of clonidine overdose

ABSORPTION/ DISTRIBUTION
- Oral bioavailability 90%
- Protein binding 46%
- V_D 2 L/kg

MOA
- Competitive antagonist at opioid receptors
- Highest affinity for MOP

EFFECTS
CVS
- Hypertension
- Ventricular arrhythmias
RS
- Pulmonary hypertension
OTHER
- Antalgesia

NALOXONE
Opioid antagonist
- Clear solution for IV use
- 0.2 or 0.4 mg/mL

DOSE
- 0.1–2 mg, titrate to effect. Onset time 2 min, duration 20 min (i.e. shorter than duration of action of morphine, so may require infusion)

METABOLISM AND EXCRETION
- Hepatic metabolism by glucuronidation
- Excreted in urine

CHEMICAL PROPERTIES
- No information

23. LOCAL ANAESTHETICS

Local anaesthetic drugs are extensively used by anaesthetists in everyday clinical practice and therefore their pharmacology makes a good SOE question incorporating both basic pharmacology and neuronal physiology. (Local anaesthetic toxicity is covered in Part 3, 'Critical incidents', Chapter 66.)

How are local anaesthetics classified?

All local anaesthetics are composed of an aromatic group linked to an amine group via an intermediate link chain. It is the nature of this link that classifies local anaesthetics as either esters or amides.

Lignocaine

Aromatic part · Amide link · Basic Amine side chain

Procaine

Aromatic part · Ester link · Basic Amine side chain

Fig. 23.1 Schematic representation of the structures of local anaesthetics

Amide local anaesthetics:
> The am*i*des all contain an '*i*' in the drug name followed by '*caine*', e.g. l*i*gnoca*i*ne, bup*i*vaca*i*ne, levobup*i*vaca*i*ne, rop*i*vaca*i*ne, pr*i*loca*i*ne and et*i*doca*i*ne.
> They are extensively bound to α_1-acid glycoprotein and albumin in the plasma. Binding decreases with a reduction in pH, so that hypoxia and acidosis can lead to toxicity.
> They undergo hepatic metabolism by hepatic amidases. Therefore, metabolism is affected in conditions resulting in reduced hepatic blood flow.
> Local anaesthetic preparations may contain the preservative sodium metabisulphite or methyl parahydroxybenzoate. These preparations should not be used for subarachnoid injection, as they have been associated with arachnoiditis.
> They are stable in solution and have a shelf-life of approximately two years.

Ester local anaesthetics:
> Examples of esters include cocaine, amethocaine and procaine.
  (A way to remember: **CAPE: C**ocaine, **A**methocaine, **P**rocaine = **E**sters)
> Undergo hydrolysis by pseudocholinesterases found principally in plasma.
> Compared to amides, esters are unstable in solution, and the incidence of hypersensitivity reactions is greater with esters, often due to the breakdown product p-aminobenzoic acid (PABA).

How do local anaesthetics exert their effects?
> Local anaesthetics act by blocking sodium channels.
> They are weak bases with a $pK_a > 7.4$. This means that they are ionised at physiological pH (7.4).
> Open sodium channel block – In the un-ionised form the local anaesthetics are lipid soluble, which allows transfer of the drug across the neuronal membrane into the axoplasm (pH 7.1), where the drug subsequently becomes ionised, blocking the sodium channels in the neuronal membrane from 'inside'. This stabilises the membrane and prevents the generation of further action potentials. Local anaesthetics bind more avidly to sodium channels that are inactivated or open, and so they are more likely to affect nerves that have a rapid firing rate. Pain and sensation nerves fire at a higher frequency than motor and so they are blocked preferentially, though all excitable membranes can be affected. This is called 'state-dependent blockade'.
> Closed sodium channel block (membrane expansion theory) – The un-ionised local anaesthetic dissolves in the neuronal membrane resulting in swelling of the neuronal membrane and consequent physical inactivation of neuronal sodium channels preventing depolarisation of the neuron.

What factors govern the potency of a local anaesthetic?
> The more lipid soluble the drug, the greater its potency, e.g. bupivacaine is seven times more lipid soluble than lignocaine and therefore more potent.

What factors govern the duration of action?
> The more protein bound the drug, the longer its duration of action, e.g. bupivacaine is 95% protein bound and has a longer duration of action than lignocaine, which is 65% protein bound.
> Addition of vasoconstrictors, such as adrenaline, also prolongs the duration of action by reducing washout of the drug into the bloodstream.

What factors govern the speed of onset?
> Speed of onset of action is closely related to the pK_a and the resulting degree of ionisation.
> Local anaesthetics with a lower pK_a (close to pH 7.4) will have a higher un-ionised fraction than those with a higher pK_a. This means that a greater proportion of the administered dose will be available to cross the neuronal membrane, and so the drug will take effect more quickly. At physiological pH (7.4), bupivacaine (pK_a 8.1) is 15% un-ionised. Lignocaine (pK_a 7.9) is 25% un-ionised and therefore has a faster onset of action.
> Clinically, bicarbonate may be added to some epidural solutions to raise the pH of the solution and therefore cause the local anaesthetic to be more un-ionised, resulting in faster onset of block.
> Infected tissue and abscesses are associated with a reduced local pH. This results in a higher fraction of the local anaesthetic becoming ionised, reducing its efficacy. Reducing efficacy further is the increased local blood flow to the infected area, causing local anaesthetic washout.

How does the rate of systemic vascular absorption of local anaesthetic agents vary?
The site of injection is important especially in terms of toxicity as the rate of systemic vascular absorption of local anaesthetic varies:
> Intercostal space > Caudal > Epidural > Brachial Plexus > Femoral > Subcutaneous

What are the salient features of the commonly used local anaesthetics?

Lignocaine:
> Amide
> Fast onset (pK$_a$ 7.9)
> Medium duration of action (70% protein bound)
> Moderate vasodilatation
> Max dose 3 mg/kg or 7 mg/kg with adrenaline

Bupivacaine:
> Amide
> Racemic mixture of R and S enantiomers
> Long duration of action (95% protein bound)
> Max dose 2 mg/kg
> Extremely cardiotoxic in overdose

Levobupivacaine:
> Amide
> S enantiomer of bupivacaine
> Long duration of action (95% protein bound)
> Less cardiotoxic in overdose than bupivacaine
> Max dose 2 mg/kg

Ropivacaine:
> Amide
> Long duration of action (94% protein bound)
> More selective sensory neuronal blockade, less motor block
> Less cardiotoxic than both bupivacaine and levobupivacaine
> Max dose 3.5 mg/kg

Prilocaine:
> Amide
> Fast onset (pK$_a$ 7.8).
> Medium duration of action (56% protein bound)
> Contained in EMLA (5% Eutectic Mixture of Local Anaesthetic – 2.5% lignocaine and 2.5% prilocaine)
> Methaemoglobinaemia can occur at high doses (due to breakdown product O-toluidine)
> Less toxic than lignocaine
> Used in intravenous regional anaesthesia (Bier's block)
> Maximum dose 6 mg/kg (9 mg/kg with felypressin)

Cocaine:
> Ester
> Short duration of action
> Profound vasoconstriction – constituent of Moffat's solution (topical)
> Blocks neuronal re-uptake 1 and stimulates CNS
> Side effects include hypertension, hallucinations, seizures and coronary ischaemia
> Max dose 3 mg/kg

24. ANTIEMETICS AND PROKINETICS

The physiology and risk factors of nausea and vomiting are covered in Study Guide 1, *Part 1, 'Physiology', Chapter 21, 'Nausea and vomiting'.*

Which receptors play a role in the stimulation of vomiting?

The vomiting centre is located within the medulla and receives afferent stimuli from multiple areas including the chemoreceptor trigger zone (CTZ), peripheral pain receptors, cerebral cortex (pain, anxiety, vision, taste), vestibular and cerebellar nuclei, and from chemoreceptors and pressure receptors in the gut. The CTZ lies close to the area postrema on the floor of the fourth ventricle, outside the blood–brain barrier. It is well placed to detect blood-borne toxins. It has many receptors including:

> Histamine (H_1)
> Muscarinic (mAChR)
> Dopaminergic (D_2)
> Serotonergic (5-HT_3)
> Opioid
> α_1 and α_2 adrenoceptors.

Stimulation of any of these receptors may ultimately lead to the activation of the vomiting centre and therefore most anti-emetic drugs act as antagonists to the receptor sites of the CTZ. As there are several receptor systems involved in the physiology of nausea and vomiting, it seems obvious that a combination of drugs acting at different receptors would have a greater antiemetic efficacy (i.e. a 'multimodal' approach).

What measures can you take to reduce the incidence of post-operative nausea and vomiting (PONV)?

PONV is a real concern to many patients presenting for surgery. The incidence ranges from 12% to 38% (risk factor dependent), and the effects of PONV can impact significantly on recovery time and hospital length of stay (and therefore cost). Strategies to minimise the risk of PONV should commence pre-operatively and continue into the post-operative period.

> **Pre-operative period:**
>   • Patients at risk of PONV should be identified during the anaesthetic assessment.
>   • Anxiolysis – benzodiazepine premedication to reduce anxiety has been shown to reduce PONV in at risk patients.
>   • Pre-hydration – oral carbohydrate containing solutions given 2 hours pre-operatively reduce PONV (this forms part of the Enhanced Recovery Programme for major gastrointestinal surgery). Keeping starvation times to a minimum and using peri-operative intravenous fluid hydration all reduce PONV.

> **Intra-operative period:**
>   - Anaesthetic agent – avoid use of nitrous oxide and, if feasible, inhalation agents for high-risk patients. As the duration of anaesthesia increases (i.e. MAC hours) so does the incidence of PONV. Total intravenous anaesthetic techniques using propofol are associated with a reduction in PONV rates.
>   - Analgesia – pain and anxiety both increase PONV and therefore good peri-operative analgesia is imperative at reducing PONV. Use regional anaesthetic techniques where possible as this can reduce opioid and volatile agent requirements. Multimodal and pre-emptive analgesic strategies (i.e. opioid reducing/sparing) also reduce PONV.
>   - Anti-emetic agents – the use of one or more anti-emetic agents reduces PONV. Each additional agent has an additive effect and can reduce the risk of PONV by 30% (so-called rule of one-third).

Give examples of anti-emetic drugs that act at the major receptor sites.

> **Histamine receptor antagonists** (e.g. cyclizine and cinnarizine):
>   - Antihistamines exert their antiemetic action at H_1 receptors within the CNS. The sedative side effect of these drugs may also contribute to their efficacy.
>   - Antihistamines are useful in the treatment of motion sickness, PONV and vestibular disorders causing vertigo.
>   - Side effects include dry mouth, urinary retention, blurred vision and sedation. Cyclizine causes tachycardia if given intravenously, and more rarely can cause extrapyramidal effects and confusion.
> **Muscarinic receptor antagonist** (e.g. hyoscine and atropine)
>   - The antimuscarinic (or anticholinergic) drugs act as competitive antagonists of muscarinic receptors at the vomiting centre and also in the gastrointestinal tract (GIT). Here, they are anti-spasmodic and decrease salivary and gastric secretions, consequently reducing gastric distension.
>   - They are the most effective therapy available for motion sickness, and are also effective for opioid-induced nausea.
>   - Side effects are predictable, and include dry mouth, blurred vision, urinary retention, tachycardia and sedation.
> **Dopaminergic receptor antagonists** (e.g. phenothiazines, metoclopramide, domperidone and butyrophenones)
>   - Phenothiazines (e.g. prochlorperazine, chlorpromazine and promethazine) act on both the dopaminergic receptors at the CTZ and the muscarinic receptors at the vomiting centre.
>   - Prochlorperazine's (Stemetil) side effects include extrapyramidal symptoms, especially in children.
>   - Chlorpromazine is mainly used in the terminally ill as its use is limited by its serious side effects that include extrapyramidal symptoms, sedation, impaired temperature regulation, increased growth hormone and prolactin release, agranulocytosis, haemolytic anaemia and leucopenia.
>   - Promethazine is also an antihistamine. It causes profound sedation, which often precludes its use as an antiemetic.
>   - Metoclopramide is a dopamine antagonist at the CTZ but also works directly on the GIT causing increased gastric motility. It is an effective antiemetic in gastrointestinal and biliary disorders. Its side effects include acute dystonic reactions (particularly oculogyric crises in young women and the very elderly), sedation, diarrhoea and neuroleptic malignant syndrome.

- Domperidone is a dopamine antagonist at the CTZ. It is of particular use in the treatment of nausea and vomiting associated with cytotoxic therapy. It does not cross the blood–brain barrier and so is relatively free of side effects. It can rarely cause GIT disturbances and hyperprolactinaemia.
- Butyrophenones (e.g. droperidol, benperidol and haloperidol) are dopamine antagonists at the CTZ. They are also mild histamine antagonists and anticholinergics. They have many side effects including extrapyramidal symptoms, neuroleptic malignant syndrome, altered temperature regulation, hypotension, tachycardia, arrhythmias and endocrine effects including weight gain and galactorrhoea.
- Droperidol is an effective antiemetic but it causes dissociation and dysphoria, which limit its use.
- Benperidol and haloperidol are prescribed for their anti-psychotic actions and are not used to treat nausea.

> **5-HT$_3$ receptor antagonists** (e.g. ondansetron and granisetron)
  - There are four types of serotonergic receptors but 5-HT$_3$ receptors are abundant at the CTZ, and are also found in the GIT.
  - The 5-HT$_3$ receptor antagonists are effective in the treatment and prevention of PONV and the nausea and vomiting associated with chemotherapy.
  - Side effects include headache, flushing, diarrhoea, constipation, drowsiness, tachycardia, bradycardia and ECG changes.

> **Steroids** (e.g. dexamethasone and methylprednisolone)
  - High doses of dexamethasone and methylprednisolone are effective in the treatment of nausea caused by cytotoxic agents and in PONV. Dexamethasone may be used alone or in combination for the prevention and treatment of PONV, but its mode of action is unclear.

> **Propofol**
  - Posseses antiemetic properties when given at sub-hypnotic doses at the end of surgery (e.g. 10–20 mg bolus for an adult) and also when used to induce and maintain anaesthesia (TIVA regime). The exact mechanism of action is unclear but it is thought to have an effect on 5-HT$_3$ receptors.

> **Benzodiazepines** (e.g. lorazepam)
  - Lorazepam has sedative, amnesic and antiemetic properties. It is used as an antiemetic during chemotherapy.
  - It is thought that lorazepam modulates central pathways involved in nausea and vomiting.

> **Neurokinin-1 receptor antagonists** (anti-NK 1, e.g. aprepitant)
  - These are currently being researched and may represent the final common pathway in the stimulation of the vomiting reflex. Blockade of NK 1 receptors is associated with broad-spectrum anti-emesis in a wide range of species.

> **Cannabinoids** (e.g. nabilone)
  - Nabilone is a synthetic cannabinoid that mimics an ingredient of cannabis. It is approved for the treatment of chemotherapy-induced nausea and vomiting and as an analgesic adjunct for neuropathic pain.
  - It causes drowsiness, dizziness, dry mouth and sometimes also psychosis.

> **Acupuncture**
  - Acustimulation to point P6 (pericardium 6, which is 2.5–5 cm proximal to the distal crease of the wrist) has been shown to reduce the incidence of PONV.
  - Studies have shown that it can provide a further 30% reduction in PONV when used in combination with ondansetron.
  - Special wrist bands that exert pressure at this point can be purchased to reduce the incidence of travel sickness.

Which drugs increase gastric motility and how do they exert their effects?

> **Metoclopramide:** This D_2 receptor antagonist also exerts prokinetic effects by stimulation of muscarinic, 5-HT_3 and 5-HT_4 receptors in the GIT. It causes relaxation of the pyloric sphincter, leads to increased peristalsis in the jejunum and duodenum, and increases stomach emptying, which may contribute to its antiemetic actions. It crosses the BBB and therefore can cause extrapyramidal side effects. Metoclopramide is often used on ICU for the treatment of gastric stasis and ileus.

> **Domperidone:** This D_2 receptor antagonist is primarily an antiemetic but it also increases gastrointestinal motility. It is used in the treatment of postprandial bloating, reflux and belching. Unlike metoclopramide, it does not cross the BBB and therefore it has minimal central side effects. The intravenous form was withdrawn following reports of significant cardiovascular arrhythmias.

> **Erythromycin:** Mimics the effect of the gut peptide motilin and acts as an agonist at the motilin receptors found mainly in the gastric antrum and proximal duodenum. It increases gastric emptying and can be used for the short-term treatment of gastroparesis. It is more effective when given orally compared with intravenously. Side effects include abdominal cramps, diarrhoea, nausea and vomiting, and rarely, tornado de pointes.

> **Neostigmine:** This acetylcholinesterase inhibitor increases the availability of acetylcholine (ACh) at the myenteric plexus, resulting in increased gut motility, salivation, gastric secretions and sphincter tone. It is occasionally used on the ICU to treat refractory constipation.

> **Cisapride:** This prokinetic agent acts at 5-HT_4 receptors enhancing ACh release at the myenteric plexus. This increases sphincter tone and peristalsis and the drug used to be prescribed for reflux oesophagitis. It has now been withdrawn in the UK because it causes long Q-T syndrome, VT, VF and torsades de pointes.

Which drugs inhibit gastric motility and how do they exert their effects?

> **Antimuscarinic agents** (e.g. atropine and hyoscine):
  • An increase in parasympathetic tone in the GIT promotes 'resting and digesting'. Antimuscarinic drugs antagonise the muscarinic M_3 receptors, decreasing GIT motility, saliva production, gastric secretions and lower oesophageal sphincter tone.

> **Opioids:**
  • Morphine and other opioids are agonists at the MOP receptors in the myenteric plexus. Stimulation of MOP receptors leads to hyperpolarisation of cells, which reduces stomach emptying, decreases gut motility and increases intestinal transit time. They also decrease gastric, biliary and pancreatic secretions. Opioids cause constipation and commonly cause nausea and vomiting by their stimulation of opioid receptors at the CTZ.

Cyclizine

ABSORPTION/
DISTRIBUTION
- Well absorbed orally
- Oral bioavailability 75%
- $t_{1/2}$ 10 hours

USES
- Antiemetic
- Ménière's disease

MOA
- Competitive antagonist at H_1 and muscarinic receptors

EFFECTS
GI
- ↑ Lower oesophageal sphincter tone
CVS
- Tachycardia
OTHER
- Pain on injection because pH of solution is 3.2
- Mild sedation

METABOLISM
AND EXCRETION
- Hepatic metabolism
- Decrease dose in liver failure
- Excreted in urine

CYCLIZINE
Antihistamine
- Tablets: 50 mg
- Solution: 50 mg/mL

DOSE
- 50 mg 8 hourly (adult)
- 1 mg/kg 8 hourly (children)

CHEMICAL PROPERTIES
- Nil

Chlorpromazine

USES
- Treatment of nausea and vomiting mostly in terminally ill (because although it is effective, its side-effects limit its use)
- Treatment of hiccoughs
- Antipsychotic

ABSORPTION/ DISTRIBUTION
- Well absorbed orally
- Significant first-pass metabolism
- Oral bioavailability 30%
- Protein binding > 90%

MOA
- Antagonises
  - D_2
  - Muscarinic
  - α_1 and α_2
  - H_1
  - 5-HT receptors
- Inhibits uptake 1

EFFECTS
CVS
- Vasodilation and hypotension
CNS
- Sedation
- Extrapyramidal side-effects (D_2 antagonist)
- Neuroleptic malignant system (rare)
- ↑ Growth hormone
- ↑ Prolactin
- Hypothermia and impaired temperature regulation
GI
- Antiemetic
- ↑ Weight
OTHER
- Agranulocytosis
- Haemolytic anaemia
- Leucopenia
- Cholestatic jaundice
- Antimuscarinic effects

CHLORPROMAZINE
Phenothiazine
- Tablets: 10/25/50/100 mg
- Syrup: 5 mg/mL
- Suppositories: 100 mg
- Solution (IM): 25 mg/mL

DOSE
- Oral: 10–50 mg 8 hourly
- IM: 25–50 mg 8 hourly
- PR: 100 mg 8 hourly

METABOLISM AND EXCRETION
- Hepatic metabolism
- Excreted in urine and bile

CHEMICAL PROPERTIES
- Nil

Domperidone

USES
• Nausea and vomiting, especially following chemotherapy

ABSORPTION/
DISTRIBUTION
• Extensive first-pass metabolism
• Oral bioavailability 15%
• Protein binding 92%
• $t_{1/2}$ 7½ hours

MOA
• Antagonises D_2 receptors
• Does not cross BBB so fewer extrapyramidal side-effects

EFFECTS
GI
• ↑ Tone of lower oesophageal sphincter
OTHER
• ↑ Prolactin secretion causing gynaecomastia and galactorrhoea

DOMPERIDONE
Butyrophenone
• Tablets: 10 mg
• Suspension: 1 mg/mL
• Suppositories: 30 mg
• Solution (IM): 12.5 mg/mL

DOSE
• 10–20 mg 8 hourly PO
• 60 mg 8 hourly PR

METABOLISM
AND EXCRETION
• Hepatic metabolism
• Excreted in faeces and urine

CHEMICAL PROPERTIES
• Nil

Metoclopramide

USES
- Antiemetic
- Prokinetic

MOA
- Antagonises D_2 receptors at chemoreceptor-trigger zone (CTZ)
- Antagonises $5\text{-}HT_3$ receptors
- Agonist at muscarinic receptors so increases gut motility

ABSORPTION/ DISTRIBUTION
- Well absorbed orally
- Significant first-pass metabolism
- Oral bioavailability 30–90%

METABOLISM AND EXCRETION
- Hepatic metabolism
- Metabolites and unchanged drug excreted in urine

METOCLOPRAMIDE
Benzamine
- Tablets/Slow release capsules: 10/15 mg
- Syrup: 1 mg/mL
- Solution: 5 mg/mL

DOSE
- 10 mg 8 hourly

CHEMICAL PROPERTIES
- Nil

EFFECTS
GI
- ↑ Tone of lower oesophageal sphincter
- ↓ Tone of pyloric sphincter
- Prokinetic
CNS
- Crosses BBB so can cause extrapyramidal side-effects
- Oculogyric crisis – usually in females < 21 years old
- Neuroleptic malignant syndrome (rare)
- Sedation
- Agitation
CVS
- Hypotension (rare)
- Tachycardia (rare)
ENDOCRINE
- ↑ Prolactin causing gynaecomastia and galactorrhoea
- Precipitates porphyria crisis

Ondansetron

USES
- Antiemetic (NB not effective for motion sickness)
- Effective in PONV & chemotherapy induced N & V (CINV)

ABSORPTION/ DISTRIBUTION
- Well absorbed orally
- Oral bioavailability 60%
- Protein binding 75%
- $t_{1/2}$ 3 hours

MOA
- Antagonises peripheral and central 5-HT$_3$ receptors

EFFECTS
GI
- Constipation
CNS
- Headache
CVS
- Bradycardia
- Flushing
- Caution in patients with risk factors for prolonged QT interval/ cardiac arrhythmias. Dose dependent prolongation of QT interval & cardiac arrhythmias including torsades de pointes. For CINV a dose limitation is now set & all doses should be diluted prior to administration in patients > 65 years.

METABOLISM AND EXCRETION
- Hepatic metabolism
- Decrease dose in liver failure
- Excreted in urine

ONDANSETRON
Carbazole
- Tablets: 4/8 mg
- Solution: 2 mg/mL

DOSE
- 4–8 mg 8 hourly (adult)
- 100 µg/kg 8 hourly (children > 2 years old)

CHEMICAL PROPERTIES
- Nil

Prochlorperazine

USES
- Nausea and vomiting
- Vertigo and motion sickness
- Psychosis
- Premedication

EFFECTS
CNS
- Extrapyramidal symptoms
- Acute dystonias and akathesia in young patients
- Mildly sedating
GI
- Cholestatic jaundice
OTHER
- Haematological abnormalities
- Skin sensitivity
- ↑ Prolactin
- Neuroleptic malignant syndrome
- Pruritis
- Antiandrogen

ABSORPTION/ DISTRIBUTION
- Variable oral absorption
- Significant first-pass metabolism
- Oral bioavailability low

MOA
- Antagonises D_2 receptors

METABOLISM AND EXCRETION
- Hepatic metabolism
- Excreted in bile and urine

PROCHLORPERAZINE
Phenothiazine

- Tablets: 3/5/25 mg
- Syrup: 1 mg/mL
- Suppositories: 5/25 mg
- Solution (IM): 12.5 mg/mL

DOSE
- 5–20 mg 8–12 hourly

CHEMICAL PROPERTIES
- Nil

25. ANTIARRHYTHMIC DRUGS

Antiarrhythmics are classified traditionally according to the Vaughn–Williams system (see Table 25.1). This system is not particularly useful as many drugs are not included (e.g. adenosine and digoxin) and many could fit into more than one category (e.g. amiodarone and sotalol). However, the examiners still expect you to know it. Many of the drugs have actions other than just their antiarrhythmic ones, and they are discussed in more detail in their relevant spider diagrams.

When answering questions on antiarrhythmics it is best to draw the graph of the nodal and myocyte action potentials to illustrate your answers.

Describe the classification of antiarrhythmic drugs.

Fig. 25.1 Cardiac myocyte action potential

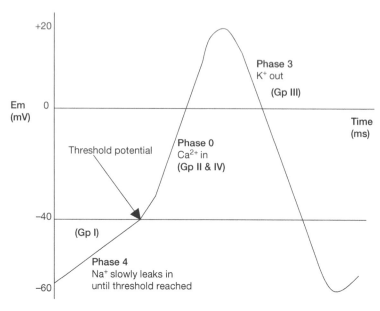

Fig. 25.2 Sinoatrial node action potential

Table 25.1 Vaughn-Williams classification of antiarrhythmics

Class	Mechanism	Drug
Ia	Blocks fast Na⁺ channels in cardiac myocytes.	Quinidine, procainamide, disopyramide
	↑ Refractory period	
Ib	Blocks fast Na⁺ channels in cardiac myocytes.	Lignocaine, phenytoin, mexiletine
	↓ Refractory period	
Ic	Blocks fast Na⁺ channels in cardiac myocytes.	Flecainide, propafenone
	No effect on refractory period	
II	β-adrenoreceptor blockade	Atenolol, propranolol, esmolol
III	K⁺ channel blockade	Amiodarone, sotalol, bretylium
IV	Ca²⁺ channel blockade	Verapamil, diltiazem

Groups II–IV refer to the class of antiarrhythmic agents that exert their effect at the various phases of the sinoatrial node action potential.

How do class I drugs exert their effects?

Refer to the cardiac myocyte AP graph (Figure 25.1):

The sodium channel blockers exert their effects by blocking fast Na⁺ channels, therefore reducing the influx of Na⁺ into cardiac myocytes and increasing the time it takes the cell to reach threshold potential. By doing this they decrease the slope of Phase 0 of the AP and decrease cardiac conduction velocity. For this reason, they are effective at abolishing re-entrant arrhythmias. These fast Na⁺ channels are not found in nodal tissue, where Phase 0 depolarisation results from the influx of Ca²⁺ ions.

Class I drugs are further sub-classified according to their effects on the refractory period (RP) of the myocyte. Class I drugs may prolong or decrease the time taken for repolarisation, and therefore the RP, by their action on the K⁺ channels responsible for Phase 3 of the AP.

How do class II drugs exert their effects?

Refer to the sinoatrial node AP graph (Figure 25.2):

β-blockers are antagonists at β adrenoceptors and so decrease sympathetic tone on the heart, which reduces the slope of Phase 4 of the AP.

β-adrenoceptors are found in nodal, conducting and myocardial tissues and are coupled, via G proteins, to Ca^{2+} channels that open when the receptor is activated. In the cardiac tissues there are relatively more β_1 than β_2 adrenoceptors, and the newer generations of β-blockers are much more cardioselective, $(\beta_1 > \beta_2)$. Blocking β adrenoceptors causes a decrease in Ca^{2+} flux into cells and so reduces the slope of Phase 0 of the AP. A decrease in Ca^{2+} influx causes:

> Decrease in heart rate (chronotropy)
> Decrease in contractility (inotropy) as less Ca^{2+} is available to the sarcomeres in the myocytes

β-blockers also inhibit the action of myosin light chain kinase and so they decrease the heart's relaxation rate (lusitropy).

How do class III drugs exert their effects?

Refer to the sinoatrial node AP graph (Figure 25.2):

Class III antiarrhythmics block K^+ channels, decreasing K^+ flux out of the cells, which delays repolarisation both in nodal tissue and in the cardiac myocytes. This decreases the slope of Phase 3 of the AP, which leads to an increase in the cells' refractory period and hence reduces its arrhythmogenicity.

How do class IV drugs exert their effects?

Refer to the sinoatrial nodal AP graph (Figure 25.2):

Class IV antiarrhythmics block L-type Ca^{2+} channels, while leaving T-, N- and P-type channels unaffected. L-type channels are widespread throughout the cardiovascular system. T-type are structurally similar to L and are present in the cardiac cells that have T-tubule systems, e.g. SA node and some vascular tissues. N-type are found in nerve cells and P in the Purkinje fibres. L-type Ca^{2+} channels are responsible for the plateau phase of the cardiac action potential. Class IV drugs decrease the slope of Phase 0 of the nodal AP, decreasing heart rate. These channels are also found in cardiac myocytes and blood vessels and decreasing Ca^{2+} flux reduces cardiac conduction velocity and contractility.

What are the main differences between verapamil and nifedipine?

Verapamil is a racemic mixture whose L isomer has a high affinity for the L-type Ca^{2+} channels at the SA and AV nodes. This results in slowing of conduction through the pacemaker cells, a decrease in heart rate and an increase in the RP. Verapamil's effect on cardiac contractility and vascular tone is less marked though it does cause some coronary artery vasodilation.

Nifedipine has little effect on the SA or AV nodes but causes a marked decrease in arterial tone. For this reason it is used for arterial spasm in coronary angiography, Raynaud's phenomenon, hypertension and angina.

SVTs can be treated with drugs from groups:	VTs can be treated with drugs from groups:
Ia	Ia
Ic	Ib
III (but not bretylium)	Ic
IV	III

Quinidine

USES
- Termination of SVTs including AF/flutter
- Termination of ventricular arrhythmias

MOA
- Class 1a antiarrhythmic
- Blocks fast Na^+ channels
  - Prolongs phase 0 of action potential
  - Increases refractory period
- ↓ Vagal tone

ABSORPTION/ DISTRIBUTION
- Oral bioavailability 75%
- Protein binding ~90%
- $t_{1/2}$ 5–9 hours

METABOLISM AND EXCRETION
- Hepatic metabolism
- Excreted in urine

QUINIDINE
Class 1a antiarrhythmic

CHEMICAL PROPERTIES
- Nil

EFFECTS
CVS
Can cause:
- Other arrhythmias, e.g. heart block, sinus tachycardia & ventricular arrhythmiast
- Hypotension

ECG
- Long PR
- Wide QRS
- Long QT and torsardes de pointes

CNS
- Cinchonism, i.e. tinnitus, blurred vision, hearing loss, headache, confusion

CAUTION!
- Displaces digoxin from binding sites causing toxicity
- Vagolytic effects can ↑ SA nodal rate and increase AV nodal conduction. In AF/flutter this can allow more impulses to reach the ventricles. Hence, preload with β-blocker/Ca^{2+} channel antagonist before treatment

Lignocaine

USES
- Local anaesthetic
- Termination of VTs

ABSORPTION/
DISTRIBUTION
- 33% ionised in blood
- Protein binding 64%
- V_D 0.7–1.5 L/kg
- $t_{1/2}$ 90–110 min

MOA
- Class 1b antiarrhythmic
- Blocks fast Na^+ channels
- ↓ Slope of Phase 0 action potential
- ↓ Refractory period
- ↓ Vagal tone

EFFECTS
TOXICITY!
Signs of toxicity:
> 4 µg/mL
- Perioral tingling
- Dizziness
- Tinnitus
- Parasthesia
> 5 µg/mL
- Altered consciousness
- Coma
- Seizures
> 10 µg/mL
- AV block
- Refractory hypotension
- Cardiac arrest
Allergy is rare

METABOLISM
AND EXCRETION
- Hepatic metabolism
- Excreted in urine (<10% unchanged)

LIGNOCAINE
Amide local anaesthetic and
Class 1b antiarrhythmic
- Routes of administration: topical/infiltration/intrathecally/ epidurally
- 1/2% clear colourless solution +/– 1:200 000 adrenaline
- Gel: 21.4 mg/mL
- Ointment: 5%
- Spray: 10%
- Aqueous solution: 4%
- EMLA cream: 2.5% lignocaine + 2.5% prilocaine

MAX DOSE
- IV 3 mg/kg or 7 mg/kg if in combination with adrenaline

CHEMICAL PROPERTIES
- Nil

Flecainide

USES
- Termination of
  - SVT
  - VT
  - WPW

MOA
- Class Ic antiarrhythmic
- Blocks fast Na^+ channels
  - Prolongs phase 0 of action potential
  - No effect on refractory period

ABSORPTION/ DISTRIBUTION
- Well absorbed orally
- Bioavailability 90%
- Protein binding 50%

EFFECTS
CVS
- May precipitate conduction disorders
- Caution with sinoatrial and atrioventricular disease
- Negative inotrope – can precipitate heart failure
OTHER
- Dizzyness
- Parasthesia
- Headache

FLECAINIDE
Amide local anaesthetic
Class 1c antiarrhythmic
- Tablets: 50/100 mg
- Solution: 10 mg/mL

DOSE
- Oral: 100–200 mg BD IV
- Loading: 2 mg/kg over 30 min (max 150 mg)
- Maintenance: 1.5 mg/kg/hr for first hour then 250 µg/kg/hr for 24 hours

METABOLISM AND EXCRETION
- Hepatic metabolism
- Active metabolites and unchanged drug excreted in urine

CHEMICAL PROPERTIES
- Nil

Amiodarone

USES
- Termination of SVT, VT, WPW (The 'domestos' of antiarrhythmics – 'kills all known arrhythmias')

MOA
- Class III antiarrhythmic but also has properties of I, II and IV
- Blocks K^+ channels, slows depolarisation, $\uparrow$ AP duration & $\uparrow$ RP

ABSORPTION/ DISTRIBUTION
- Very poorly absorbed
- Protein binding 95%
- V_D 2–70 L/kg
- $t_{1/2}$ 20–100 days!

METABOLISM AND EXCRETION
- Hepatic metabolism
- Excreted by biliary tract, lacrimal glands and skin

AMIODARONE
Class III antiarrhythmic
- Tablets: 100/200 mg
- Solution: 150 mg clear colourless – dilute in 5% dextrose

DOSE
- IV loading: 5 mg/kg over 1 hour, into large vein
- Maintenance: 15 mg/kg/day infusion (usually patients given 300 mg loading + 900 mg over 24 hours)
- Oral: 200 mg t.d.s. for 1 week, reducing to BD for 1 week, reducing to od there onwards

CHEMICAL PROPERTIES
- Highly irritant, give into large vein

EFFECTS
CVS
- Prolonged QT
- Hypotension
- Bradycardia
RS
- Pneumonitis 10% affected after 3 years, 10% associated mortality
CNS
- Peripheral neuropathy and myopathy (rare)
- Corneal micro deposits halos and blurred vision. Regular sight tests essential. Reversible effect
GI
- Metallic taste
- Cirrhosis, jaundice, hepatitis – check LFTs regularly
SKIN
- Photosensitivity
- 'Slate-grey' skin
THYROID
- Hypo/hyperthyroidism
- Affects iodide absorption and conversion from T4 to T3
DRUG INTERACTIONS
- Highly protein-bound and so can displace other drugs bound to protein, e.g. digoxin, and precipitate toxicity.
- Avoid with other drugs which prolong QT (tricyclics, thiazides) can cause torsades de pointes.
- Caution with AV node blockers, e.g. β-blockers can cause heart block.

USES
- To slow rate of AF and flutter
- Inotrope in cardiac failure

MOA
- Binds to and inhibits Na^+/K^+ATPase pump. This causes rise in intracellular $[Na^+]$. This decreases extrusion of Ca^{2+} by Na^+/Ca^{2+} exchange pump, because this relies on high concentration gradient of Na^+ across cell membrane (which is reduced).
- ↑ intracellular Ca^{2+} causes ↑ contractility
- ↓ intracellular K^+ causes ↓ conduction in SA & AV node, slowing HR
- Increases vagal tone, so ↑ AV conduction time

EFFECTS
CVS
Arrhythmias and conduction abnormalities:
- Premature ventricular contraction
- Bigeminy
- AV block – all types
- Junctional rhythm
- Atrial/ventricular tachycardia

ECG
- Long PR (toxicity)
- 'Inverted tick' (toxicity)
- Flat T wave (at therapeutic level)
- Short QT (at therapeutic level)

OTHER
- Anorexia
- Nausea and vomiting
- Diarrhoea
- Headache
- Lethargy
- Visual disturbances of red-green perception
- Rashes
- Eosinophilia
- Gynaecomastia

Plasma levels:
- ↑ by amiodarone, erythromycin, captopril
- ↓ by antacids, phenytoin, metoclopramide

ABSORPTION/ DISTRIBUTION
- Oral bioavailability > 70%
- Protein binding 25%
- V_D 5–10 L/kg
- $t_{1/2}$ 35 hours, ↑↑↑ in renal failure

METABOLISM AND EXCRETION
- Minimal hepatic metabolism
- Excreted unchanged in urine

DIGOXIN
Glycoside extracted from foxglove leaves (*digitalis lanata*)
- Tablets: 62.5–250 µg
- Colourless solution: 100–250 µg/mL

DOSE
- Loading: 500 µg followed by 500 µg or 250 µg 6 hours later (depending on patient's size)
- Maintenance: 62.5–500 µg/day
- Therapeutic range: 1–2 µg/L

TOXICITY
- **TOXIC** at [plasma] > 2.5 µg/L serious effects not usually seen at < 10 µg/L
- > 30 µg/L fatal
- Treat bradycardia with atropine or pacing
- Treat ventricular arrhythmias with phenytoin
- 'Digibind' antidote available (IgG antibody fragments against digoxin, bind and the complex is removed by kidneys), but very expensive. Use if > 20 µg/L, life threatening arrhythmias, uncontrolled hyperkalaemia
- Digibind can cause anaphylaxis

Verapamil

USES
- Termination of SVT (most common use), AF and atrial flutter.
- Prophylaxis of angina
- Hypertension

ABSORPTION/ DISTRIBUTION
- Well absorbed (90%) but extensive first-pass metabolism
- Oral bioavailability 25%
- Protein binding 90%
- V_D 3–5 L/kg
- $t_{1/2}$ 3–7 hours

MOA
- Class IV antiarrhythmic
- Block L-type Ca^{2+} channels so ↓ slope of nodal AP
- ↓ Ca^{2+} influx so ↓ conduction velocity and contractility
- Coronary artery dilation

EFFECTS
CVS
- May precipitate VF or VT in WPW
- CCF in patients with poor LV function
- Caution with β–blockers/digoxin/ halothane – severe bradycardia
- Hypotension (may be desirable)

OTHER
- Cerebral vasodilatation

VERAPAMIL
Calcium channel antagonist
- Tablets: 40–240 mg
- Solution: 2.5 mg/mL

DOSE
- Oral: 240–480 mg /day in 3 divided doses
- IV: 5–10 mg over 30 s, titrate to effect
- Peak effect: 3–5 min
- Duration: 10–20 min

METABOLISM AND EXCRETION
- Hepatic metabolism subject to zero order kinetics
- Both active metabolites and unchanged drug excreted in urine

CHEMICAL PROPERTIES
- Nil

β-Blockers

ABSORPTION/ DISTRIBUTION
- Varying lipid solubility of different agents
- Low lipid solubility, e.g. atenolol = poorly absorbed from gut
- Higher lipid solubility, e.g. metoprolol = well absorbed, but cross BBB and ↑ CNS side-effects
- Variable protein binding

USES
- Hypertension
- Angina and MI
- Tachycardias
- Obtund reflex hypertension during laryngoscopy, e.g. esmolol
- In phaeochromocytoma – pre-op stabilisation
- HOCM
- Anxiety
- Glaucoma
- Migraine prophylaxis

EFFECTS
CVS
- Negative inotrope and chronotrope so:
  - ↑ Time in diastole and coronary artery perfusion
  - ↓ Cardiac oxygen requirements BUT, may worsen performance of failing ventricle
- ↓ BP
  - ↓ HR and CO
  - ↓ Renin secretion by β_1 inhibition at juxtaglomerular apparatus BUT: beware in peripheral vascular disease as inhibition of β_2 receptors causes some constriction which may further compromise circulation in peripheries.

RS
- Bronchospasm, worse in susceptible patients so give cardioselective drugs in asthma/COPD and give test dose of short acting drug, e.g. esmolol/metoprolol

CNS
- Cross BBB can cause:
  - Hallucinations
  - Nightmares
  - Depression
  - Fatigue
  - ↓ Intra-ocular pressure

GI
- Dry mouth
- GI upset

METABOLIC
Non-selective agents can:
- ↑ Resting BM in diabetics
- Mask symptoms of hypoglycaemia (sweating, tachycardia, etc.)
- ↑ Triglycerides and ↓ HDL

MOA
- All competitive antagonists at β adrenoceptor
- Some have intrinsic sympathomimetic activity
- Varying receptor affinity (see box below)

METABOLISM AND EXCRETION
- Low lipid solubility = minimal hepatic metabolism and excreted unchanged in urine
- High lipid solubility = hepatic metabolism

β-BLOCKERS
(Class II antiarrhythmic)

RECEPTOR SELECTIVITY
Aim to block β_1 but not β_2 receptors.
'Cardioselective' drugs:
- Atenolol
- Esmolol (ultra-short acting)
- Metoprolol (short acting)
- Bisoprolol
- Carvedilol
NB all will act on β_2 if dose high enough

Adenosine

USES
- To differentiate between SVT (rate slows) and VT (rate doesn't slow)
- If tachyarrhythmia is re-entrant, it may terminate it
- To differentiate between atrial fibrillation and flutter, by slowing ECG trace for analysis

MOA
- Binds to adenosine (A1) receptors coupled with K^+ channels that open, to hyperpolarised membrane
- A1 receptors only found in sinoatrial and atrioventricular nodes so adenosine selectively decreases conduction velocity in the nodes (negative dromotropic effect)
- Also decreases cAMP mediated catecholamine stimulation of ventricles (negative chronotropic effect)

ABSORPTION/ DISTRIBUTION
- $t_{1/2} < 10$ s

METABOLISM AND EXCRETION
- Deamination in plasma and red blood cells

ADENOSINE
Naturally occurring purine nucleoside
- Colourless solution: 3 mg/mL

DOSE
- Give incremental doses at 1 min intervals until desired effect achieved 6 mg/12 mg/ 12 mg
- Give as fast bolus into large vein

EFFECTS
CVS
- No clinically significant effects on BP when given as described

OTHER
- ↑Pulmonary vascular resistance
- SOB, flushing and chest discomfort
- Bronchospasm in asthmatics
- Sense of impending doom. (Patients genuinely feel like they're going to die. Warn them of this and support them through the feeling. It only lasts a few seconds.)

CHEMICAL PROPERTIES
- Nil

26. ANTIHYPERTENSIVE AGENTS

What are the major categories of antihypertensive drugs and what are their mechanism of actions?

$$MAP = CO \times SVR$$
$$CO = SV \times HR \text{ (SV depends on preload, contractility and afterload)}$$

Antihypertensive agents will produce their effect by modulating cardiac output (CO), systemic vascular resistance (SVR) or both. The easiest way to categorise antihypertensive agents is according to their site of action:

Heart:
> **β-Blockers** – Competitive antagonists at β-adrenoceptors with varying degrees of receptor selectivity. Negative inotropic and chronotropic effects reduce CO while antagonism of the renal $β_1$ adrenoceptors reduces sympathetically mediated release of renin.
  - **Atenolol, esmolol and metoprolol** – Cardioselective (i.e. act only on $β_1$ adrenoceptors at normal doses).
  - **Propranolol** – Non-cardioselective (i.e. acts at both $β_1$ and $β_2$ adrenoceptors).
  - **Labetalol** – Non-cardioselective and has antagonistic action at $α_1$-adrenoceptors (ratio of $α_1$: β blockade depends on the route of administration: oral = 1:3 and IV = 1:7).

Blood vessels:
> **Directly acting vasodilators** – Produce NO, which acts on G-protein-coupled receptors activating guanylate cyclase and increasing intracellular cGMP levels to cause vasodilatation.
  - **Sodium nitroprusside and hydralazine** – Produce vasodilatation of both arterial and venous vessels. Arterial vasodilatation reduces SVR while venous vasodilatation increases venous capacitance and reduces preload.
  - **Glyceryl trinitrate and isosorbide mononitrate** – Produce vasodilatation of primarily the venous vessels. This increases venous capacitance and reduces preload.
> **Indirectly acting vasodilators** – Reduce SVR and preload by various mechanisms.
  - **Calcium channel blockers** (e.g. amlodipine) – Antagonists at L-type calcium channel located in vascular smooth muscle.
  - **α-Blockers** (e.g. prazosin) – Antagonists at $α_1$-adrenoceptors causing vasodilatation of both arterial and venous vessels.
  - **Potassium channel activators** (e.g. nicorandil) – Activators of ATP-sensitive K^+ channels within arterioles causing hyperpolarisation, reduced intracellular Ca^{2+} levels and hence arteriolar vasodilatation. Venous vessels are also relaxed by activation of guanylate cyclase by the nitrate moiety within nicorandil.
  - **Magnesium** – This is a natural antagonist to calcium.

Kidney:
> **Diuretics** – Reduce plasma volume (which reduces preload and CO) and some produce arteriolar vasodilatation reducing SVR (e.g. thiazide and loop diuretics). *See* Chapter 27, 'Diuretics'.
> **Agents affecting the renin–angiotensin–aldosterone system** (*See* later)
>   • Angiotensin-converting enzyme inhibitors, ACEI (e.g. ramipril)
>   • Angiotensin II receptor antagonists (e.g. losartan)

Central nervous system:
> **Centrally acting drugs** (e.g. clonidine and methyldopa) – Stimulate central inhibitory presynaptic α_2-adrenoceptors causing reduced noradrenaline release and hence reduced centrally mediated sympathetic outflow.
> **Ganglion blockers** (e.g. trimetaphan) – Competitive antagonists at nACh receptors located in parasympathetic and sympathetic ganglia.

Briefly explain the renin–angiotensin–aldosterone system (RAAS).

RAAS system is intricately involved in the regulation of blood pressure. Renin is released from the juxtaglomerular apparatus in response to low renal perfusion, reduced Na^+ at the macula densa or sympathetic stimulation via renal β_1 adrenoceptors. Renin converts angiotensinogen, which is produced by the liver, into angiotensin I. Angiotensin I is then converted into angiotensin II in the lung via the action of angiotensin-converting enzyme (ACE). Angiotensin II produces a multitude of effects including peripheral vasoconstriction, aldosterone release from the adrenal cortex, increased thirst sensation, and increased ADH (also known as vasopressin) and ACTH release from the hypothalamo–pituitary axis.

What are some of the more common side effects of antihypertensive agents?

> **β-Blockers** – Unwanted side effects come from antagonism of β_2 adrenoceptors, which may cause bronchospasm and peripheral vasoconstriction. Hence these agents are best avoided in patients with COPD and peripheral vascular disease.
> **Vasodilators** – Vasodilatation of the capacitance vessels can cause postural hypotension while vasodilatation of cerebral vessels can lead to headaches.
> **Diuretics** – Loop and thiazide diuretics can both lead to hyponatraemia, hypokalaemia, hypomagnesaemia and hypochloraemic alkalosis due to their action on renal electrolyte reabsorption. Loop diuretics can also cause ototoxity leading to deafness while thiazide diuretics can cause hyperuricaemia and precipitate gout. Owing to the risk of hypokalaemia, these agents should be used cautiously with digoxin.
> **ACEI** – Under normal conditions angiotensin II maintains renal perfusion by altering the calibre of the efferent arteriole at the glomerulus. However, in the presence of an ACEI this mechanism is lost and renal perfusion pressure may fall, leading to renal failure in those individuals who already have impaired renal circulation. Hence these agents are contraindicated in renal artery stenosis. Some patients may experience a persistent cough due to increased bradykinin, which is normally degraded by ACE.

Nimodipine

USES
• Reduction of vasospasm
  following subarachnoid
  haemorrhage (SAH)
• Migraine

ABSORPTION/
DISTRIBUTION
• Well absorbed orally
• Significant first-pass
  metabolism
• Oral bioavailability up to 28%
• Protein binding 98%
• V_D 0.94–2.3 L/kg

MOA
• Competitive antagonist
  at slow calcium
  channels causing
  decreased influx of Ca^{2+}
  into cells
• Relatively selective for
  cerebral arterioles

EFFECTS
CVS
• ↓ SVR and BP at
  > 2 mg/hr
CNS
• Increased cerebral blood
  flow secondary to
  vasodilatation
• Headache
• Vertigo

METABOLISM
AND EXCRETION
• Hepatic metabolism
• Excreted in urine

NIMODIPINE
Dihydropyridine calcium
channel antagonist
• Tablets: 30 mg
• Solution: 200 µg/mL

DOSE
• Oral: 60 mg 6x/day for SAH
• IV: 1–2mg/hr

CHEMICAL PROPERTIES
• Nil

Nifedipine

USES
- Angina
- Hypertension
- Reduction of vasospasm during coronary angiography
- Raynaud's phenomenon

EFFECTS
CVS
- ↓ SVR and BP
- ↑ HR and ↓ contractility
- ↑ CO
- ↑ Coronary oxygen requirements
- Sublingual administration can cause precipitous fall in BP
- Flushing
CNS
- Small increased cerebral blood flow secondary to vasodilatation
- Headache
- Vertigo
RS
- Inhibits hypoxic pulmonary vasoconstriction
OTHER
- Negatively inotropic effects of nifedipine are additive with those of the volatiles, especially isoflurane. Use together with caution
- ↓ MAC
- Prolong effects of neuromuscular blocking drugs

ABSORPTION/ DISTRIBUTION
- Well absorbed orally
- Oral bioavailability 60%
- Protein binding 95%
- $t_{1/2}$ 5 hours

MOA
- Competitive antagonist at slow calcium channels causing decreased influx of Ca^{2+} into cells

NIFEDIPINE
Calcium channel antagonist
- Capsules: 5–10 mg
- Tablets: 10–60 mg
- Onset in: 15–20 min

DOSE
- 10–20 mg 8 hourly

METABOLISM AND EXCRETION
- Hepatic metabolism
- Excreted in urine

CHEMICAL PROPERTIES
- Nil

Captopril

USES
- Hypertension
- Reduction of progression of diabetic nephropathy
- Post MI, to improve ventricular remodelling

EFFECTS
CVS
- ↓ SVR and BP
- Afterload ↓ > preload
- First-dose hypotension – give test dose at night

RENAL
- Angiotensin II (AII) autoregulates renal perfusion pressure by altering arteriolar tone. ACEI reduce plasma AII, which can cause ↓ perfusion and ∴ renal failure
- So, contraindicated in renal artery stenosis

METABOLISM
- ↓ Aldosterone leads to ↑ renin secretion
- ↑ K^+ (as less exchanged for Na^+) so avoid using with K^+ sparing diuretics

OTHER
- Can cause refractory hypotension with anaesthesia – some advise omitting for 24 hours prior to surgery
- Dry cough results from ↑ serum bradykinin
- Angio-oedema (more common in Afro-Caribbean patients)
- Agranulocytosis
- Thrombocytopenia
- Rash, ulcers
- Caution with NSAIDs – increase chance of renal failure

ABSORPTION/ DISTRIBUTION
- Well absorbed orally
- Oral bioavailability 75%
- Protein binding 30%
- V_D 0.61–0.79 L/kg
- $t_{1/2}$ 1.9 hours

MOA
- Angiotensin converting enzyme (ACEI) preventing conversion of angiotensin I to II

CAPTOPRIL
ACE Inhibitor
- Tablets: 12.5/25/50 mg

DOSE
- Oral: 12–50 mg/day, starting at 6.25 mg and titrating up

METABOLISM AND EXCRETION
- Hepatic metabolism
- Excreted in urine, 50% unchanged

CHEMICAL PROPERTIES
- Nil

Losartan

USES
- Hypertension
- To reduce progression of diabetic nephropathy, independent of its antihypertensive effect
- Used when dry cough of ACE inhibitors unacceptable
- Not usually first line, as more expensive than ACE inhibitor

ABSORPTION/ DISTRIBUTION
- Well absorbed orally
- Significant first-pass metabolism
- Oral bioavailability 30%
- Protein binding 99%
- V_D 0.61–0.79 L/kg
- $t_{1/2}$ 2 hours

MOA
- Antagonist at angiotensin II receptors

EFFECTS
CVS
- ↓ SVR and BP
- Afterload ↓ > preload
- first-dose hypotension – give test dose at night
RENAL
- Angiotensin II (AII) autoregulates renal perfusion pressure by altering arteriolar tone and so antagonists can cause ↓ perfusion and renal failure
- So, contraindicated in renal artery stenosis
OTHER
- Can cause refractory hypotension with anaesthesia – some advise omitting for 24 hours prior to surgery
- Does not block actions of ACE, therefore no increase in bradykinins and no cough
- Caution with NSAIDs – increased chance of renal failure

LOSARTAN
Substituted imidazole
AII receptor antagonist
- Tablets: 25/50 mg

DOSE
- 50–100 mg/day

METABOLISM AND EXCRETION
- Hepatic metabolism
- Excreted in urine and bile

CHEMICAL PROPERTIES
- Nil

Nicorandil

USES
• Angina – treatment and prophylaxis

MOA
• Activates K⁺channels, i.e. opens them. K⁺ flows out of cell hyperpolarising the membrane
• This closes Ca^{2+} channels, reducing Ca^{2+} concentration and decreasing contractility and cardiac work
• Causes venous relaxation and reduction of preload by donating nitric oxide to cells. This increases cGMP and reduces Ca^{2+} (*see* GTN, next page, for full explanation)

EFFECTS
CVS
• ↓ Preload
• ↓ LVEDP
• ↓ Cardiac work
• Flushing
CNS
• Vertigo
• Headache
OTHER
• Nausea and vomiting
• Angio-oedema
• Hepatic dysfunction

ABSORPTION/ DISTRIBUTION
• Well absorbed orally
• Protein binding 0%
• $t_{1/2}$ 1 hour

METABOLISM AND EXCRETION
• Hepatic metabolism
• Excreted in urine and bile

NICORANDIL
Nicotinamidoethyl nitrate
K⁺ channel activator
• Tablets: 10/20 mg

DOSE
• 10–30 mg 12 hourly

CHEMICAL PROPERTIES
• Nil

Glyceryl Trinitrite

USES
- Prophylaxis/treatment of angina
- CCF and pulmonary oedema
- MI, ACS
- Hypertension
- Patch over vein to maintain dilation, e.g. for peripheral feeding

ABSORPTION/ DISTRIBUTION
- Well absorbed orally
- Significant first-pass metabolism
- Oral bioavailability 5%
- Protein binding 60%
- V_D 0.04–2.9 L/kg

MOA
- GTN broken down to liberate nitric oxide (NO)
- NO increases cGMP, so Ca^{2+} uptake into smooth muscle is reduced leading to vasodilation

EFFECTS
CVS
- ↓ SVR and BP
- Predominantly venodilatation so ↓ preload
CNS
- ↑ ICP causing headache
OTHER
- Tolerance develops to patches, so have 'patch-free period' each day
- No significant tolerance develops to IV infusion
- Methaemoglobinaemia (rare)

GLYCERYL TRINITRATE (GTN)
Organic Nitrate
- Tablets: 300/600 μg S/L
- Buccal: 2/5 mg prn
- Spray: 400 μg/spray S/L prn
- Patch: 5–10 mg/24 hours
- Solution: 5 mg/mL infused at 1–10 mg/hr titrated to BP
- Sublingually – effective in 3 min lasts 1 hour

METABOLISM AND EXCRETION
- Hepatic metabolism to di/mononitrites
- Excreted in urine

CHEMICAL PROPERTIES
- Explosive, so remove patches before cardioversion

Clonidine

USES
- Hypertension
- Agitation and anxiety on ICU
- Adjunct in neuroaxial anaesthesia
- Migraine
- Analgesia

ABSORPTION/DISTRIBUTION
- Well absorbed orally
- Oral bioavailability 100%
- Protein binding 20%
- V_D 2l L/kg
- $t_{1/2}$ 9–18 hours

MOA
- Agonist at presynaptic α_2 receptors, so decreasing sympathetic tone
- In spinal cord they increase release of endogenous opiates
- Effective within 10 min

EFFECTS
CVS
- ↓ SVR and BP
- Rebound hypertension if stopped suddenly
CNS
- Sedation, anxiolysis
- ↓ MAC
RENAL
- Diuresis? result of ADH inhibition
HAEMATOLOGICAL
- No increase in platelet aggregation, despite their surface α_2 receptors
OTHER
- ↓ Post-operative analgesia requirements

CLONIDINE
- Tablets: 100/250/300 μg
- Solution: 150 μg/mL

DOSE
- Oral: 50–600 μg 8 hourly
- IV: 75–300 μg 8 hourly

METABOLISM AND EXCRETION
- Hepatic metabolism
- Excreted in urine, 50% unchanged

CHEMICAL PROPERTIES
- Nil

Sodium Nitroprusside

USES
• Hypertension

MOA
• Broken down to liberate nitric oxide (NO)
• NO increases cGMP, so Ca^{2+} uptake into smooth muscle is reduced leading to vasodilation

ABSORPTION/ DISTRIBUTION
• Not absorbed orally
• $t_{1/2}$ 10 min

SODIUM NITROPRUSSIDE
• Red/brown powder 50 mg/vial
• Reconstitute with 5% dextrose

DOSE
• 0.5–6 µg/kg/min titrate to effect

METABOLISM AND EXCRETION
• Metabolised two ways:
  1 Reacts with sulphydryl groups on plasma proteins
  2 Hydrolysis in red blood cells to liberate NO + 5 cyanide (CN^-) ions + methaemoglobin.
• Of the 5 CN^-s:
  • 1 CN^- reacts with Hb $\rightarrow$ cyanomethaemoglobin
  • 4 CN^- enter plasma, and of these:
  • 3 CN^- react with thiosulphate $\rightarrow$ thiocyanate
  • 1 CN^- reacts with hydroxy-cobalamin $\rightarrow$ cyanocobalamin

CHEMICAL PROPERTIES
• Biodegrades in sunlight so use opaque giving sets or wrap normal ones in tin foil

EFFECTS
CVS
• Arteriolar dilation, $\downarrow$ SVR and BP
• Venodilatation, $\downarrow$ preload
• $\downarrow$ LVEDP
• $\downarrow$ Myocardial O_2 consumption
RS
• $\downarrow$ Hypoxic pulmonary vasoconstriction, so give O_2 to reduce shunt
CNS
• $\uparrow$ ICP
• Dizziness
ENDOCRINE
• $\uparrow$ Catecholamines
• $\uparrow$ Renin
TOXICITY
• Cyanide irreversibly inhibits respiration by binding to cytochrome oxidase
• Signs:
  • Tachycardia, arrhythmias
  • Hyperventilation
  • Sweating
  • Rising SVO_2
  • Metabolic acidosis
• More common in
  • Liver/renal failure
  • Vit B_{12} deficiency
OTHER
• Nausea and vomiting
• Muscle twitching
• Tachyphylaxis

USES
- Hypertension
- Pregnancy induced hypertension and pre-eclampsia

EFFECTS
CVS
- ↓ SVR and BP
- Postural hypotension (rare)
- Rebound hypertension if stopped suddenly

CNS
- Sedation
- Vertigo
- Depression, nightmares (uncommon)

RENAL
- Urine darkens on standing due to oxidation of methyldopa and its metabolites

GI
- Constipation
- Impaired liver function with long-term use
- Hepatic necrosis reported

HAEMATOLOGICAL
- Direct Coombe's test + in 10–20%
- Haemolytic anaemia
- Thrombocytopenia (rare)
- Leucopenia (rare)

OTHER
- Decreases MAC
- Hypersensitivity to drug can cause myocarditis
- Gynaecomastia

ABSORPTION/ DISTRIBUTION
- Variable oral absorption
- Undergoes first-pass metabolism
- Variable oral bioavailability 8–60%
- Protein binding < 20%

MOA
- Metabolised to α -methyl noradrenaline, which is an α_2 agonist
- This is taken up into nerve terminals in CNS, and when released decreases sympathetic tone

METHYLDOPA
Phenylalanine derivative
- Tablets: 125/250/500 mg
- Solution: 50 mg/mL

DOSE
- 0.5–3 g/day in 2–3 doses

METABOLISM AND EXCRETION
- Hepatic metabolism
- Excreted in urine, 50% unchanged

CHEMICAL PROPERTIES
- Nil

Prazosin

USES
- Hypertension
- Benign prostatic hypertrophy
- Raynaud's phenomenon
- Treatment of nightmares associated with post-traumatic stress disorder

ABSORPTION/
DISTRIBUTION
- Oral bioavailability 50–80%
- Protein binding 92%
- V_D 0.5–0.89 L/kg

MOA
- Highly selective α_1 competitive antagonist

EFFECTS
CVS
- α_1 blockade
- Vasodilation and ↓ BP
- Little reflex tachycardia
GU
- Relaxes bladder sphincters
SIDE-EFFECTS
- Profound orthostatic hypotension
- Syncope
- Nasal congestion
- Fatigue
- Headache
- Vertigo
- Nausea and vomiting
  These side-effects may be pronounced after the first dose ('first-dose effect'), but may resolve with continued use

PRAZOSIN
Quinazoline derivative
- Tablets: 0.5/1/2/5 mg

DOSE
- 0.5 mg t.d.s. increasing to max of 20 mg/day

METABOLISM
AND EXCRETION
- Hepatic metabolism
- Excreted in bile

CHEMICAL PROPERTIES
- Nil

Phenoxybenzamine

USES
- Hypertensive emergencies, especially caused by
  - Phaeochromocytoma
  - Cocaine
- Reynaud's phenomenon
- Complex regional pain syndrome, because it modulates the sympathetic nervous system

MOA
- Non-selective irreversible α-blocker
- New receptors must be synthesised to overcome drug effect
- Blockade of α_2 receptors increases the amount of noradrenaline released
- Partial agonist at 5-HT$_2$ receptors

ABSORPTION/ DISTRIBUTION
- Oral bioavailability ~ 25%
- Protein binding 50%
- $t_{1/2}$ 24 hours

EFFECTS
CVS
- α_1 blockade
- Vasodilation and $\downarrow$ BP
- Reflex tachycardia causes $\uparrow$ CO
- α_2 blockade enhances noradrenaline release causing $\uparrow$ HR and $\uparrow$ CO

CNS
- Sedation
- Meiosis
- Convulsions with rapid infusion
- Dizziness

OTHER
- Little effect on GI/renal blood flow
- Dry mouth
- Impotence
- Contact dermatitis

PHENOXYBENZAMINE
α-blocker
- Capsules: 10 mg
- Solution: 50 mg/mL

DOSE
- Oral: 10–60 mg per day in divided doses
- IV: 10–40 mg over 1 hour Lasts for 3–4 days

METABOLISM AND EXCRETION
- Hepatic metabolism
- Excreted in urine and bile

CHEMICAL PROPERTIES
- Nil

Phentolamine

USES
- Hypertensive emergencies, especially caused by:
  - Phaeochromocytoma
  - Cocaine
  - MAOI reactions with tyramine
- Inject into corpus callosum to facilitate erection in impotence
- Used in diagnosis and treatment of complex regional pain syndrome as this has an element of sympathetic mediation

ABSORPTION/ DISTRIBUTION
- Oral bioavailability 20%
- Protein binding 50%
- $t_{1/2}$ 15 min

MOA
- Competitive α blocker
- 3x higher affinity for α_1 than α_2
- β receptor agonist activity
- Anti-serotonergic activity

EFFECTS
CVS
- α_1 blockade
  - Vasodilation and $\downarrow$ BP
  - $\uparrow$ Coronary artery perfusion
  - $\downarrow$ Pulmonary artery pressure
- α_2 blockade
  - Enhances noradrenaline release causing $\uparrow$ HR and $\uparrow$ CO
- Marked nasal congestion, use topical vasoconstrictors if planning nasal instrumentation
RS
- $\uparrow$ VC and $\uparrow$ FEV$_1$
- $\uparrow$ Secretions
- Prevents bronchospasm caused by histamine release
GI
- GI motility
- Salivation
- Gastric acid secretions
OTHER
- Insulin secretion can cause hypoglycaemia

PHENTOLAMINE
Imidazoline
- Pale yellow solution: 10 mg/mL

DOSE
- 1–5 mg titrate to effect
- Onset in 1–2 min
- Offset in 5–20 min

METABOLISM AND EXCRETION
- Extensively metabolised
- 10% excreted unchanged in urine

CHEMICAL PROPERTIES
- Nil

β-Blockers

ABSORPTION/ DISTRIBUTION
- Varying lipid solubility of different agents
- Low lipid solubility, e.g. atenolol = poorly absorbed from gut
- Higher lipid solubility, e.g. metoprolol = well absorbed, but cross BBB and ↑ CNS side-effects
- Variable protein binding

USES
- Hypertension
- Angina and MI
- Tachycardias
- Obtund reflex hypertension during laryngoscopy, e.g. esmolol
- In phaeochromocytoma – pre-op stabilisation
- HOCM
- Anxiety
- Glaucoma
- Migraine prophylaxis

EFFECTS
CVS
- Negative ionotrope and chronotrope so:
  - ↑ Time in diastole and ↑ coronary artery perfusion
  - ↓ Cardiac oxygen requirements
  BUT, may worsen performance of failing ventricle
- ↓ BP
  - ↓ HR and CO
  - ↓ Renin secretion by β_1 inhibition at juxtaglomerular apparatus
  BUT: beware in peripheral vascular disease as inhibition of β_2 receptors causes some constriction which may further compromise circulation in peripheries

RS
- Bronchospasm, worse in susceptible patients, so give cardioselective drugs in asthma/COPD and give test dose of short-acting drug, e.g. esmolol/metoprolol

CNS
- Cross BBB can cause:
  - Hallucinations
  - Nightmares
  - Depression
  - Fatigue
  - ↓ Intra-ocular pressure

GI
- Dry mouth
- GI upset

METABOLIC
Non-selective agents can:
- ↑ Resting BM in diabetics
- mask symptoms of hypoglycaemia (sweating, tachycardia, etc)
- ↑ Triglycerides and ↓ HDL

MOA
- All competitive antagonists at β adrenoreceptor
- Some have intrinsic sympathomimetic activity
- Varying receptor affinity (*see box below*)

METABOLISM AND EXCRETION
- Low lipid solubility = minimal hepatic metabolism and excreted unchanged in urine
- High lipid solubility = hepatic metabolism

β BLOCKERS
(Class II antiarrhythmic)

RECEPTOR SELECTIVITY
Aim to block β_1 but not β_2 receptors
'Cardioselective' drugs:
- Atenolol
- Esmolol (ultra-short acting)
- Metoprolol (short acting)
- Bisoprolol
- Carvedilol
NB all will act on β_2 if dose high enough

27. DIURETICS

Draw a nephron and indicate where diuretic drugs exert their effects.

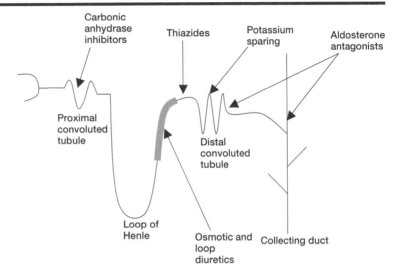

Fig. 27.1 Schematic representation of the nephron indicating the sites of action of various diuretic agents

How does mannitol exert its effects?

> Mannitol is a sugar alcohol solution, which works as an osmotic diuretic.
> The drug has a molecular weight of 182 Daltons and so is freely filtered by the glomerulus but not reabsorbed.
> It increases the osmolality of the filtrate and so water follows the drug to be excreted.
> Osmotic activity occurs mainly at proximal convoluted tubule and loop of Henle.

What is the major indication for using mannitol?

Mannitol is used primarily in the treatment of raised intracerebral pressure (ICP). It reduces ICP by:

> Decreasing the formation of CSF.
> Decreasing plasma volume and thereby encouraging water to move out of the brain, reducing oedema. Mannitol does not cross the intact blood–brain barrier. However, if the membrane is disrupted, mannitol can cross it and worsen oedema by drawing water with it. Hence, unless a patient is actively coning, it should only be used on the advice of a neurosurgeon.
> It is free radical scavenger and so may afford some additional neuroprotection.

Can mannitol be used repeatedly?

No, mannitol is used to 'buy time' until raised ICP can be treated definitively. The dose cannot be repeated indefinitely, as it will cause an unacceptable rise in serum osmolality and circulatory overload. With repeated dosing it will eventually cross the blood–brain barrier and cause a rise in ICP.

What are the side effects of the thiazides and loop diuretics?

Please refer to the appropriate spider diagram for this answer.

How are diuretics used in renal failure?

Diuretics do not reverse renal failure, but they can be used to control its symptoms. The use of diuretics, particularly loop diuretics, reduces:

> Hypertension, mediated by decreased sodium excretion and water retention
> Congestive cardiac failure caused by circulatory overload
> Oedema.

Large doses of the drugs may be needed as their efficacy is decreased in the face of low renal blood flow, reducing delivery to their target organ. It may be necessary to give the drugs by continuous infusion and to combine various diuretics to achieve optimum results.

Furosemide

USES
- CCF
- Peripheral and pulmonary oedema
- To force diuresis in acute and chronic renal failure

MOA
- Act mainly on thick ascending limb of loop of Henle, and less so on early distal convoluted tubule
- Inhibit reabsorption of Na^+ and Cl^-
- This impairs counter-current multiplier system
- Medulla becomes less hypertonic so less water reabsorbed

ABSORPTION/ DISTRIBUTION
- Both well absorbed orally
- Bioavailability = Frusemide – 65% Bumetanide – 95%
- Protein binding >95%

FUROSEMIDE
(and also bumetanide)
Loop diuretic

METABOLISM AND EXCRETION
- Excreted mostly unchanged in urine

CHEMICAL PROPERTIES
- Nil

EFFECTS

CVS
- Arteriolar vasodilation causes ↓ SVR and ↓ preload

RENAL
- ↑ Renal blood flow
- ↑ GFR

BIOCHEMISTRY
- ↓ K^+
- ↓ Cl^- ⎤ Hypochloraemic
- ↓ H^+ ⎦ alkalosis
- ↓ Na^+
- ↓ Mg^{2+}
- ↑ Ca^{2+} (less common than thiazides)
- ↑ Uric acid causes gout (less common than with thiazides)

METABOLIC
- Hyperglycaemia (less common than with thiazides)
- ↑ Cholesterol and triglycerides – though they return to baseline with long-term treatment

OTHER
- Ototoxicity – rapid IV injection can cause deafness, higher risk in patients in renal failure or on aminoglycosides

INTERATIONS
- Raise serum lithium levels

Bendroflumethiazide

USES
- Hypertension
- Heart failure

ABSORPTION/
DISTRIBUTION
- Well absorbed orally
- Effective in 90 min
- Lasts 18–24 hours

MOA
- Act on early distal convoluted tubule
- Inhibit reabsorption of Na^+ and Cl^-
- ↑ Na^+ and Cl^- excretion and ∴ ↑ H_2O excretion

METABOLISM
AND EXCRETION
- Hepatic metabolism to active compounds
- Metabolites and unchanged drug (30%) excreted in urine

BENDROFLUMETHIAZIDE
Thiazide diuretics
- Tablets: 2.5/5 mg

DOSE
- 2.5–5 mg od PO

CHEMICAL PROPERTIES
- Nil

EFFECTS
CVS
- ↓ BP as ↓ circulating volume

RENAL
- ↓ Renal blood flow
- ↓ GFR

BIOCHEMISTRY
- ↓ K^+
- ↓ Cl^-
- ↓ Na^+
- ↓ Mg^{2+}
- ↓ H^+
- ↑ Ca^{2+}
- ↑ Uric acid causing gout

METABOLIC
- ↓ Glycogenesis
- ↓ Insulin secretion
- ↑ Glycogenolysis
- ↑ Cholesterol and triglycerides
  So, use with caution in diabetics

HAEMATOLOGY
- Blood dyscariasis including:
  - Anaemia – aplastic and haemolytic
  - Leucopenia
  - Agranulocytosis
  - Thrombocytopenia

OTHER
- Impotence
- Rash
- Photosensitivity
- Pancreatitis

INTERATIONS
- Metolazone shows synergism when used with loop diuretics
- Effects antagonised by NSAIDs

Amiloride

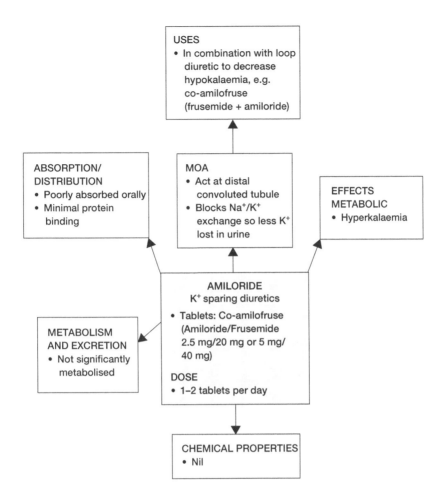

USES
- In combination with loop diuretic to decrease hypokalaemia, e.g. co-amilofruse (frusemide + amiloride)

ABSORPTION/ DISTRIBUTION
- Poorly absorbed orally
- Minimal protein binding

MOA
- Act at distal convoluted tubule
- Blocks Na^+/K^+ exchange so less K^+ lost in urine

EFFECTS METABOLIC
- Hyperkalaemia

AMILORIDE
K^+ sparing diuretics
- Tablets: Co-amilofruse (Amiloride/Frusemide 2.5 mg/20 mg or 5 mg/ 40 mg)

DOSE
- 1–2 tablets per day

METABOLISM AND EXCRETION
- Not significantly metabolised

CHEMICAL PROPERTIES
- Nil

Spironolactone

USES
- Ascites
- Nephrotic syndrome
- Conn's syndrome (primary hyperaldosteronism)

MOA
- Acts at distal convoluted tubule and collecting ducts
- Competitive antagonist of aldosterone
- Aldosterone stimulates reabsorbtion of Na^+ in exchange for K^+
- NB limited diuresis as Na^+ reabsorbtion stimulated by aldosterone only accounts for 2% of total water reabsorbed

EFFECTS
BIOCHEMISTRY
- ↑ K^+
- ↑ Na^+
HORMONAL
- Gynaecomastia in men
- Irregular menstruation due to anti-androgenic effects
OTHER
- Nausea and vomiting
- ↓ Response to vasopressors
- ↑ Response to cardiovascular depressants

ABSORPTION/ DISTRIBUTION
- Oral bioavailability 70%
- Protein binding > 90%

SPIRONOLACTONE
Aldosterone antagonist
- Tablets: 25/50/100 mg

DOSE
- 100–400 mg/day

METABOLISM AND EXCRETION
- Hepatic metabolism
- Excreted in urine

CHEMICAL PROPERTIES
- Nil

Acetazolamide

USES
- Weak diuretic
- Mountain sickness (prophylaxis and treatment)
- Glaucoma

MOA
- Acts at proximal convoluted tubule
- Non-competitive inhibitor of carbonic anhydrase (CA)
- CA catalyses:
  $CO_2 + H_2O \rightleftharpoons H_2CO_3 \rightleftharpoons H^+ + HCO_3^-$
- Affects Na^+ exchange for H^+ in PCT so, fewer H^+ ions generated for excretion
- This causes alkaline urine & mild metabolic acidosis which counteracts the respiratory alkalosis associated with ascending to altitude

EFFECTS
RS
- $\uparrow$ RR in response to $\uparrow$ CO_2

CNS
- $\downarrow$ Intra-ocular pressure by $\downarrow$ rate of aqueous humour production
- $\downarrow$ ICP by $\downarrow$ rate of CSF production

GI
- $\downarrow$ Gastric secretions
- $\downarrow$ Pancreatic secretions

RENAL
- Mild diuresis
- $\downarrow$ Excretion of uric acid

OTHER
- Hyperchloraemic metabolic acidosis and alkaline urine as H^+ excretion decreased and bicarbonate not reabsorbed

ABSORPTION/ DISTRIBUTION
- Oral bioavailability 100%
- Protein binding 70–90%
- $t_{1/2}$ up to 6 hours

METABOLISM AND EXCRETION
- Hepatic metabolism
- Excreted in urine

ACETAZOLAMIDE
Carbonic anhydrase inhibitor
- Tablets: 250 mg
- Clear colourless solution: 500 mg/vial

DOSE
- Oral: 250 mg – 1 g/day in divided doses orally
- IV: 250 mg – 1 g 4 hourly

CHEMICAL PROPERTIES
- Nil

Mannitol

USES
- To reduce raised intracranial pressure
- To force diuresis in major vascular surgery (this is no longer in vogue)

MOA
- Freely filtered by glomerulus and not reabsorbed (Mol weight 182 Da)
- Water follows mannitol as osmolality of filtrate is increased

ABSORPTION/ DISTRIBUTION
- Given IV
- $t_{1/2}$ 100 min

EFFECTS
CVS
- Initial ↑ in circulating volume – take care in patients with CCF
RENAL
- ↑ Renal blood flow
CNS
- ↓ ICP
- NB unable to cross intact BBB, but following head injury it may cross and then draw fluid into the brain, worsening ICP. So, give with caution, under guidance of neurosurgeons unless in life-threatening situation
OTHER
- Allergy, though rare
- Free radical scavenger – thought to be neuroprotective
- Dose cannot be repeated indefinitely as causes rise in serum osmolality, circulatory overload, ultimately will cross BBB and cause ↑ ICP

MANNITOL
Osmotic diuretic
- 10–20% clear colourless sugar alcohol solution

DOSE
- 0.5–1 g/kg bolus over 20 min

METABOLISM AND EXCRETION
- Not significantly metabolised
- Freely filtered at glomerulus

CHEMICAL PROPERTIES
- Nil

28. NON-STEROIDAL ANTI-INFLAMMATORY DRUGS

How do NSAIDs exert their effects?

Non-steroidal anti-inflammatory drugs (NSAIDs) exert their effects by inhibiting the action of the enzyme cyclo-oxygenase (COX) and therefore reducing the production of the inflammatory prostanoids, as shown below:

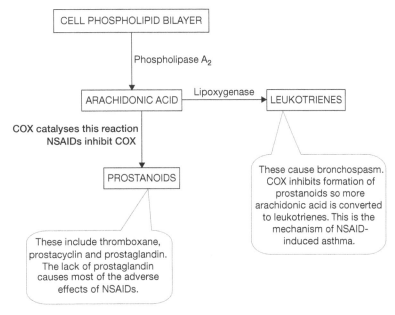

Fig. 28.1 Pathway for prostaglandin and leukotriene synthesis

Describe the distribution of cyclo-oxygenase.

There are two types of COX when discussing NSAIDs: COX 1 and COX 2.

> **COX 1** (constitutive) is found in most cells.
> **COX 2** (inducible) is undetectable in most normal tissue but found in abundance in macrophages and other cells of inflammation.
> • COX 2 catalyses the formation of inflammatory mediators and is therefore the enzyme that needs to be inhibited in order to decrease pain and inflammation. In theory, if COX 2 could be inhibited without affecting COX 1, symptoms would be improved with minimal or no side effects. In practice, this is not the case as COX 2 inhibitors still show the side-effect profile of non-specific agents.
> **COX 3** discovered in 2002, it is an isoenzyme most likely to be a CNS variant of COX 1. It is the site of action of paracetamol.

What are the main actions of prostacyclin and thromboxane?

> **Prostacyclin** is a vasodilator and prevents formation of platelet plug in primary haemostasis.
> **Thromboxane** is produced by platelets. It is a vasoconstrictor and a potent platelet aggregator.

These prostanoids are in fine balance in health.

Describe the main actions of prostaglandins.

Prostaglandins – nine different receptors result in varied actions, e.g.:
> PGE_2 – ↓ gastric acid secretion, ↑ gastric mucous secretion
> PGI_2 – vasodilatation, platelet aggregation
> $PGF_{2\alpha}$ – uterine contraction, bronchoconstriction.

Classify the NSAIDs.

> NSAIDs may be classified according to their structure:
>   • Acetylsalicylic acids, e.g. aspirin
>   • Phenylacetic acids, e.g. diclofenac
>   • Carboacetic acids, e.g. indomethacin
>   • Propionic acids, e.g. ibuprofen
>   • Enolic acids, e.g. piroxicam
> NSAIDs may also be classified according to their inhibition of cyclo-oxygenase:
>   • Non-selective COX inhibitors, e.g. aspirin, diclofenac, ibuprofen
>   • Selective COX 2 inhibitors, e.g. parecoxib.

What are the indications for use of NSAIDs?

> NSAIDs are used therapeutically for their anti-inflammatory and analgesic effects. In the management of acute pain, NSAIDs have an opioid-sparing effect.
> Aspirin compared to the other NSAIDs has a unique anti-platelet action, which is used therapeutically in the prevention of arterial thrombosis (myocardial infarction and cerebrovascular accident).

What are the main contraindications to the use of NSAIDs?

> Relative contraindications to NSAIDs include renal impairment, history of gastrointestinal bleeding, heart failure, hypertension, coagulation defects.
> Absolute contraindications include proven hypersensitivity to aspirin or any NSAIDs.
> Assess the hydration status of the patient before prescribing NSAIDs. There is a risk of precipitating renal failure if NSAIDs are administered to patients who are dehydrated.
> NSAIDs may enhance the effects of warfarin.
> NSAIDs may worsen asthma in 10–20% of patients; they are contraindicated if aspirin or any other NSAIDs have precipitated attacks of asthma, although this occurs rarely in children.
> Aspirin should not be given to children under 12 years for analgesia or children under 15 years as an antipyretic because of the risk of Reye's syndrome (aspirin-induced liver failure secondary to mitochondrial dysfunction).

What are the main side effects of NSAIDs?

The more an NSAID blocks COX 1, the greater is its tendency to cause peptic ulceration and promote bleeding. Selective COX 2 inhibitors cause less bleeding and fewer ulcers than other NSAIDs but certain drugs in this group have been associated with an increased incidence of thrombotic complications, especially myocardial infarction (rofecoxib was withdrawn in 2004 because of an increased incidence of myocardial infarction).
The following list summarises the main side effects of NSAIDs:

> NSAID-induced exacerbation of asthma (approximately 10–20% of asthmatics affected). The mechanism is thought to involve increased production of bronchoconstricting leukotrienes.

> Gastrointestinal bleeding – NSAIDs reduce circulating prostaglandins that are essential in maintaining gastric mucosal integrity.
> Acute kidney injury may be induced by NSAIDs in vulnerable patients, e.g. pre-existing renal dysfunction, diabetics, elderly or dehydrated patients. The mechanism involves reduced levels of prostacyclin, which are required to maintain renal perfusion.
> Platelet dysfunction – related to reduced thromboxane production. This is seen only with the non-specific COX inhibitors, not with the selective COX 2 inhibitors.

Paracetamol

USES
- Analgesia
- Antipyretic

ABSORPTION/
DISTRIBUTION
- Absorbed in small bowel
- Oral bioavailability 80%
- Protein binding 10%

MOA
- Central action via COX 3 inhibition which is associated with ↓ brain PGE_2 levels?
- Modulates endogenous cannabinoid system

EFFECTS
CVS
- IV solution can cause hypotension and bradycardia if given rapidly
CNS
- Analgesia
- Antipyretic
OTHER
- Rash
- Idiopathic thrombocytopenia
- Analgesic nephropathy
- Toxic in OD

METABOLISM
AND EXCRETION
- Hepatic metabolism mainly to glucuronide and sulphate metabolites (30%)
- Actively excreted in urine, small amount unchanged
- 10% metabolised by P450 system to N-acetyl-p-amino benzoquinoneimine (NAPQI) = TOXIC
- Genetic polymorphism of enzymes determines how much NAPQI is produced
- In normal doses, NAPQI is rapidly conjugated by glutathione and its harmless products excreted in urine
- Once glutathione is exhausted, NAPQI accumulates causing liver failure
- To treat OD – assess ABCD and make appropriate intervention. Give oral methionine (enhances glutathione synthesis) and/or IV N-acetylcysteine (parvolex), which is hydrolysed to a precursor of glutathione

PARACETAMOL
NSAIDs
- Tablets: 500 mg
- Suppositories: 125/500 mg and 1 g
- Solution: 1 g in 100 mL
DOSE
- Adults: 1 g 6 hourly
- Children: first dose 15–30 mg/kg followed by 15 mg/kg 6 hourly Max 90 mg/kg/24 hourly

CHEMICAL PROPERTIES
- Para-aminophenol

Aspirin

USES
- Analgesia
- Anti-inflammatory
- Anti-platelet in MI/CVA, etc.

MOA
- Pro-drug
- Irreversible COX 1 inhibitor, modifies action of COX 2
- ↑ Affinity for COX 1 at low dose
- Selectively inhibits production of TXA_2 in platelets and ∴ inhibits aggregation

ABSORPTION/DISTRIBUTION
- Absorbed mainly in small bowel
- 85%PPB

METABOLISM AND EXCRETION
- Hepatic and intestinal metabolism by ester hydrolysis to salicyclic acid (active metabolite)
- Further conjugated to salicyluric acid
- (inactive metabolite)
- First-order kinetics in low dose, becoming zero order in overdose
- Excreted in urine

ASPIRIN
Salicyclic acid derivative NSAIDs
- Tablets: 75 and 300 mg

DOSE
- Angina and stroke prophylaxis: 75 mg od
- Post MI and thrombotic stroke 300 mg as one-off dose, then continue with 75 mg od
- Analgesia: 300–900 mg 6 hourly 300 mg
- Max dose 4 g/24 hourly

CHEMICAL PROPERTIES
- Salicylate
- Weak acid, pK_a 3.0
- Poorly ionised in acidic environment of stomach. ↑ pH & larger surface area of small intestine cause aspirin to be absorbed rapidly.

EFFECTS
RS
- 20% of asthmatics sensitive to NSAIDs which can cause bronchoconstriction

GI
- ↑ Risk of GI bleeding and ulceration because inhibition of prostaglandin (PG) synthesis causes ↓ mucosal protection
- Hepatotoxic causing transaminitis

RENAL
- Inhibition of PGs and prostacyclin causes local hypoxia and ↓ renal perfusion

CVS
- ↓ Endoperoxidases and thromboxane A_2 ∴ ↓ platelet aggregation and ↓ vasoconstriction, ∴ cardioprotective
- NB effects on platelet irreversible. New platelets must be synthesised to reverse effect
- Fluid retention can precipitate heart failure

DRUG INTERACTIONS
- Care with warfarin – NSAIDs are highly protein bound and so may displace warfarin
- May ↑ lithium levels

OTHER
- Toxic in overdose
- Reye's syndrome in children

Diclofenac

ABSORPTION/
DISTRIBUTION
- Well absorbed by all routes
- Significant first-pass metabolism
- Oral bioavailability 60%
- 99.5% PPB, mainly to albumin so may displace oral anticoagulants
- V_D 0.12–0.17 L/kg

USES
- Analgesia
- Anti-inflammatory

MOA
- Inhibits cyclo-oxygenase (COX)
- Equal effect on COX 1 and 2

EFFECTS
RS
- 20% of asthmatics are sensitive to NSAIDs
GI
- As for aspirin but less GI upset
RENAL
- Inhibition of prostaglandins and prostacyclins causes local hypoxia and↓ renal perfusion
CVS
- Reversible inhibition of platelet function, little effect on bleeding time
OTHER
- Affects neutrophil function
- Renin and aldosterone concentration reduced by up to 70%
- Risk of thrombosis

DICLOFENAC
Phenylacetic acid derivative
NSAIDs
- Tablets: 25/50 mg
- Suppositories: 12.5/25/50/100 mg
- Solution: 25 mg/mL
- Topical gel

DOSE
- Adult: 50 mg 8 hourly
- Child: 1 mg/kg 8 hourly

METABOLISM
AND EXCRETION
- Hepatic metabolism
- Excreted in bile

CHEMICAL PROPERTIES
- Nil

29. ANTIBIOTICS

What is 'antimicrobial stewardship'?

This refers to a coordinated programme that promotes the appropriate prescribing and use of antimicrobials (including antibiotics) in order to reduce microbial resistance, decrease the spread of infection caused by multi-drug-resistant organisms and improve patient outcomes. In 2014, NICE published a quality standard for infection prevention and control that included antimicrobial stewardship.

What are the main principles of good antibiotic prescribing?

In order to help prevent the development of bacterial resistance, it is important to prescribe antibiotics according to the principles of antimicrobial stewardship, which include:

> Prescribe antibiotics only when clinically indicated.
> Collect specimens for culture (e.g. blood, urine) prior to starting therapy.
> Prescribe antibiotics according to local guidelines and seek microbiology advice if needed.
> Choose correct class of antibiotic that would be effective against suspected organism.
> Use targeted, narrow-spectrum agents where possible.
> If broad-spectrum therapy commenced, de-escalate as soon as possible based on microbiology-sensitivity data.
> Ensure correct duration of treatment (start and stop dates).
> Ensure correct dose (adjust for weight, renal function, liver function and if on renal replacement therapy).
> Switch intravenous agents to oral preparation promptly.
> Source control where applicable (e.g. drain collections).
> Ensure surgical prophylaxis compliance to reduce surgical site infection (ideally antibiotics should be administered 30 minutes prior to skin incision, they should be given before tourniquet is inflated and re-dose if 1500 mL blood loss or duration of surgery >4 hours).

What is concentration-dependent and time-dependent killing?

In order to answer this you need to understand a few pharmacokinetic concepts:

> **Minimum inhibitory concentration (MIC)** – lowest concentration of antibiotic required to completely inhibit growth of a particular bacterium *in vitro*.
> **Minimum bactericidal concentration (MBC)** – lowest concentration of antibiotic required to kill a particular bacterium *in vitro*.

When evaluating antibiotic efficacy, there are three important pharmacokinetic parameters:

- Peak serum level (C_{max})
- Trough serum level (C_{min})
- Area under the serum concentration–time curve (AUC)

Integrating these pharmacokinetic parameters with the MIC gives three pharmacokinetic (PK)/pharmacodynamic (PD) indices that quantify the activity of an antibiotic:

- Peak/MIC ratio – this is C_{max} divided by the MIC.
- T > MIC (time above MIC) – this is the percentage of a dosage interval in which the serum level exceeds the MIC.
- 24-h AUC/MIC ratio – this is determined by dividing the 24-h AUC by the MIC.

> **Concentration-dependent killing**, e.g. aminoglycosides – the ideal dosing regimen for these antibiotics maximise **concentration**, because the higher the concentration, the more extensive and the faster is the degree of killing. Therefore, the 24-h AUC/MIC ratio and the Peak/MIC ratio correlate best with antibiotic efficacy.

> **Time-dependent killing**, e.g. β-lactams – the ideal dosing regimen for these antibiotics maximise the **duration** of exposure. The T > MIC is the best predictor of antibiotic efficacy.

How do antibiotics exert their effects?

Antibiotics are drugs used to inhibit (bacteriostatic) or kill (bacteriocidal) bacteria. Bacteriostatic drugs require the aid of host defences to clear tissues of the infecting microorganism. If these defences are compromised (e.g. agranulocytosis) or impaired locally at the site of infection (e.g. cardiac vegetation in endocarditis), the residual pathogen resumes growth after stopping the bacteriostatic drug and the infection relapses. Their mode of action can be classified as shown in Figure 29.1.

Which factors should be considered when administering gentamicin?

> Aminoglycoside antibiotics such as gentamicin are used to treat urinary and biliary tract infections, endocarditis and septicaemia.
> They work by binding irreversibly to the 30 S subunit of the bacterial ribosome and inhibiting bacterial protein synthesis. This leads to bacterial cell death.
> These agents are administered intravenously or intramuscularly, as they are not absorbed enterally.
> At high plasma concentrations aminoglycosides can cause ototoxicity and nephrotoxicity.
> The dose of gentamicin is 3–5 mg/kg/day and can be given in divided doses every eight hours. Blood samples are taken 1 hour after the administered dose ('peak' plasma concentration) and/or just before a dose ('trough' plasma concentration). 'Peak' plasma gentamicin levels should be 5–10 mg/L and 'trough' levels should be less than 2 mg/L.
> An alternative, once-daily regime is used in some departments. Here, the full gentamicin dose is prescribed as a single dose and the frequency of administration is adjusted according to the 'trough' gentamicin levels using a nomogram, e.g. the Urban Craig nomogram.

In which patient groups should gentamicin be used with caution?

> Gentamicin should be used with caution during pregnancy as it can cross the placenta and cause fetal ototoxicity.
> Aminoglycosides are not metabolised, instead they are excreted unchanged by the kidneys, primarily by glomerular filtration. Therefore the dose and/or frequency of administration should be altered in renal failure. Renal function should be quantified using the creatinine clearance, which can be estimated using the Cockcroft and Gault formula.
> Aminoglycosides can potentiate the action of non-depolarising muscle relaxants or cause recurrence of the blockade produced by these agents. They cause this effect by interfering with calcium entry into the presynaptic terminal of the motor axon, thereby preventing the release of acetylcholine from the presynaptic vesicles. This drug interaction can even cause a neostigmine-resistant block, which can be antagonised by the use of calcium salts. Because of this effect on neurotransmission, aminoglycosides are contraindicated in patients with myasthenia gravis.

Cockcroft and Gault formula to estimate creatinine clearance (CrCl):

$$CrCl = \frac{140-\text{Age (Years)} \times \text{Weight (kg)}}{72 \times \text{serum creatinine (μmol/L)}} \times (0.85 \text{ only if female})$$

Describe the structure of penicillin.

> The basic structure comprises a thiazolidine ring nucleus attached to a β-lactam ring.
> The β-lactam ring has an amino-acid side chain, which varies between different types of penicillin and determines their main antibacterial and pharmacological properties.
> Other antimicrobial agents belonging the β-lactam group of antibiotics include:

  • Cephalosporins
  • Monobactams
  • Carbapenems.

Describe the mechanism of action of penicillin.

> Penicillins are bactericidal antibiotics that inhibit bacterial cell wall synthesis.
> The β-lactam ring binds to bacterial cell wall proteins and inhibits the formation of peptidoglycan cross-links. These cross-links are essential for maintaining bacterial cell wall stability and without them the wall is weakened, resulting in cytolysis and cell death due to osmotic pressures.
> The resultant build-up of peptidoglycan precursors stimulates the bacterial release of enzymes, which auto-digest the bacterial cell wall.

What is the spectrum of clinical use?

> Penicillins are active against most Gram-positive organisms and some Gram-negative cocci.
> They are not very effective against Gram-negative bacilli.
> They can be divided into categories depending on their spectrum of action:

  • Narrow spectrum, e.g. benzylpenicillin
  • β-lactamase resistant, e.g. flucloxacillin
  • Broad spectrum, e.g. ampicillin
  • Anti-pseudomonal, e.g. piperacillin

What is the effect of probenecid on penicillin?

Probenecid is a renal tubular blocking agent. It inhibits the tubular secretion of penicillin and usually increases penicillin plasma levels (up to 2- to 4-fold elevation in plasma concentrations has been demonstrated).

How does resistance to penicillins develop?

Inappropriate use of antibiotics and poor prescribing play a vital role in propagating antibiotic resistance. There are several mechanisms by which bacteria develop resistance to penicillins:

> **Drug inactivation** – bacterial production of β-lactamase leads to hydrolysis of the β-lactam ring.
> **Alteration of penicillin binding proteins** – this prevents the antibiotics from binding onto the bacterial cell wall.
> **Alteration of bacterial cell wall permeability** – this prevents antibiotics from penetrating the cell wall.

What are the major side effects of the penicillins?

> **Hypersensitivity** due to an allergy to the basic structure of the β-lactam group of the antibiotics. Therefore, up to 10% of patients allergic to penicillin will suffer cross-reactivity if given another antibiotic containing a β-lactam group. Hypersensitivity reactions occur in 10% of the population while anaphylaxis occurs in approximately 0.01%.
> Gastrointestinal disturbances.
> **Encephalopathy** in patients with renal failure.
> **Rash**, especially when ampicillin is administered to patients with infectious mononucleosis.

How do penicillins and aminoglycosides act synergistically?

Penicillins weaken the bacterial cell wall by inhibiting cell wall synthesis and this enables the aminoglycosides to penetrate the cell and inhibit bacterial protein synthesis intracellularly.

Fig. 29.1 Mode of action and classification of antibiotics

30. ANTICOAGULANTS

What types of heparin do you know?

Naturally occurring heparin
> A highly sulphated glycosaminoglycan carbohydrate weighing between 3000 and 50000 Daltons.
> It is produced by basophils and mast cells.

Unfractionated heparin (UFH)
> Synthetic agent weighing between 5000 and 25000 Daltons.
> It binds to and potentiates the action of antithrombin III 1000-fold.
> Activated antithrombin III inhibits thrombin and other serine proteases that promote blood clotting.

Low molecular weight heparin (LMWH), e.g. enoxaparin, dalteparin, tinzaparin
> Newer drugs weighing between 2000 and 8000 Daltons.
> LMWHs do not target antithrombin, but instead directly inhibit factor Xa.

The dose of both LMWH and UFH are calculated in units of activity rather than weight. One unit of activity is the amount of a preparation required to keep 1 mL of cat's blood fluid for 24 hours at 0 °C.

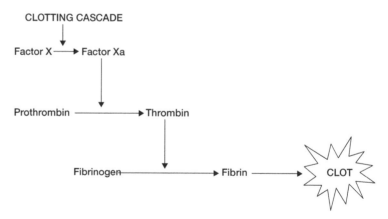

Fig. 30.1 The final common pathway of clotting.

What are the differences between the unfractionated (UFH) and low molecular weight heparins (LMWH)?

In order to inactivate thrombin, the heparin molecule must be able to bind both the antithrombin III molecule and the thrombin molecule. To do this, it must have a size greater than 18 saccharide ternary units. Smaller molecules, therefore, are only able to inhibit the activity of other proteases such as factor Xa.

Table 30.1   Comparison of unfractionated and low molecular weight heparins

	UFH	LMWH
Xa inhibition	+	+++
Protein binding	50%	10%
t½	30–150 min (dose dependent)	2–3× longer for equivalent dose
Monitoring	APTT	Anti-Xa. Not routinely monitored.
Administration	Monitored infusion	Once daily (or BD).
Bioavailability (s.c. dose)	40%	90%

How is heparin used clinically?

> **UFH:**
> * As an infusion to prevent the propagation of deep vein thrombosis (DVT) and pulmonary emboli (PE)
> * During cardiopulmonary bypass to reduce clotting of blood in contact with bypass circuit
> * During extracorporeal membrane oxygenation (ECMO) to prevent clotting in the circuit
> * During vascular surgery to prevent newly inserted stent occlusion
> * Twice daily subcutaneous dose for thrombosis prophylaxis.

Its half-life is only around 1 hour and so UFH must be given continuously by infusion. It is common practice to give a bolus of 5000 IU followed by an infusion based on the patient's weight. The patient's activated partial thromboplastin time (APTT) is measured 6 hours following the start of the infusion, and the dose is adjusted to keep the APTT at 1.5–2× normal. Because of its short half-life, the anticoagulant effects of UFH are quickly lost once the infusion is stopped. This can prove useful, e.g. if bleeding becomes a problem, or if the patient needs to go to theatre.

> **LMWH:**
> * As a twice-daily subcutaneous injection to prevent the propagation of DVT and PE
> * As a twice-daily subcutaneous injection to prevent clot propagation in acute coronary syndrome
> * Once-daily subcutaneous dose for thrombosis prophylaxis.

Because of its longer half-life, LMWH can be given once or twice daily depending on the indication.

How is heparin therapy monitored?

APTT measures the activity of the intrinsic clotting cascade (factors VIII, IX, XI and XII) and the final common pathway and is therefore prolonged by UFH. Hence, we measure APTT to monitor and alter heparin infusions appropriately.

LMWH inhibits mainly factor Xa and therefore does not affect the APTT. Usually no monitoring is required but anti-factor Xa levels can be measured as needed.

What are the side effects of heparin therapy?

> **Haemorrhage:**
> - Heparin is given subcutaneously to avoid intramuscular haematoma. It can cause fatal haemorrhage if given in overdose. Its dose should be reduced in patients with renal failure, in whom it can accumulate. UFH, but not LMWH, can be reversed with protamine (dose 1mg reverses 100IU heparin).

> **Non-immune thrombocytopenia:**
> - Occurs after approximately 4 days of therapy.
> - Platelets recover spontaneously without cessation of heparin.

> **Heparin-induced thrombocytopenia (HIT):**
> - This immune-mediated process usually takes around 5 days to develop, though prior exposure to heparin can cause an accelerated course.
> - IgG antibodies are made against heparin after it binds to platelet factor 4 (PF4).
> - These antibodies attach themselves to the heparin PF4 complex and go on to bind and activate platelets. Consequently, thrombi are formed throughout the vascular tree and the platelet count falls. HIT can result in fatal PEs, limb ischaemia and stroke.
> - In suspected HIT heparin should be discontinued and blood sent to the lab for a 'HIT screen'. Alternative anticoagulation should be used.

> **Hypotension:**
> - Can follow rapid bolusing of a large dose.

> **Other:**
> - Osteoporosis following long-term administration.
> - Alopecia.

What are the advantages of LMWH?

> It only requires once or twice daily dosing.
> It does not need monitoring.
> It is less likely to cause HIT (though it can still do so) and non-immune-mediated thrombocytopenia.

How does warfarin exert its anticoagulant effect?

Warfarin, a coumarin-based anticoagulant, is primarily indicated in the treatment of deep vein thrombosis, atrial fibrillation in patients at risk of embolisation and patients with mechanical prosthetic heart valves. It exerts its anticoagulant effect by inhibiting the synthesis of the vitamin K-dependent clotting factors (II, VII, IX and X). Anticoagulant effect is monitored via the international normalised ratio (INR). It takes at least 48 hours to achieve its clinical effect, which is why a heparin-based anticoagulant is often started at the same time if an immediate effect is needed.

Which drugs may potentiate the action of warfarin?

Warfarin is extensively protein bound (>95%). Therefore any drug that competes for the protein binding site, or any condition that reduces protein binding, will potentiate the activity of Warfarin. NSAIDs and simvastatin if administered concurrently with warfarin compete for the plasma protein binding sites, leading to warfarin displacement and increased warfarin anticoagulant effect.

There are also various drugs that affect the metabolism of warfarin such as metronidazole, macrolides and alcohol. All of these reduce its metabolism, raise the INR and increase the risk of bleeding.

Antibiotics that affect the vitamin K-producing gut flora will also increase the effect of warfarin.

What other factors can potentiate the action of warfarin?

Diet – food stuffs and supplements can increase the effect of warfarin such as St John's wort, ginger and ginseng.

Thyroid status will also affect warfarin, hypothyroidism reducing it effect.

Protein binding: as well as other drugs competing for binding sites, there are other factors that will reduce the protein binding of warfarin. Changes in plasma pH such as in severe sepsis will alter the tertiary structure of proteins and reduce binding sites. Reduced production of proteins such as in severe liver disease or old age will reduce binding.

Pregnancy – warfarin is contraindicated in pregnancy due to its teratogenic effects on the fetus (it can cause cleft lip and palate formation) and the risk of maternal bleeding. This risk is increased by the progressively reduced protein binding of warfarin through the pregnancy.

Describe the treatment of overdose of warfarin.

The main adverse effect of warfarin overdose is bleeding. Major bleeding should be managed using an 'ABC' approach. Specific treatment includes stopping the warfarin, administration of vitamin K (10 mg IV), administration of prothrombin complex concentrate e.g. beriplex (which contains factors II, VII, IX and X) or alternatively administration of 15 mL/kg of fresh frozen plasma, although the latter is falling out of favour because of the attendant risks.

What other anticoagulants do you know?

Rivaroxaban

Rivaroxaban is a direct factor Xa inhibitor that can be taken orally as a once-daily dose.

It has the advantage over warfarin in that it has a wide therapeutic window with a rapid onset of action. It therefore does not need dose adjustment or monitoring.

Dabigatran

Dabigatran is a direct thrombin inhibitor that can be given orally. It has a similar clinical effectiveness to warfarin but like rivaroxaban it does not need monitoring. Its major drawback is that there is no way to reverse its effect.

How can anticoagulants be reversed?

Protamine sulphate

Heparin's action can be reversed using protamine sulphate (as opposed to protamine). It is a highly positive molecule so forms strong ionic complexes with the highly negative heparin molecules reducing the activity of heparin and markedly increasing its elimination.

Care must be taken with its administration, as allergic reactions are common particularly in those with fish allergies, diabetics (insulin often contains protamine) and vasectomised men (sperm contains protamine).

Warfarin's action can be reversed by giving intravenous vitamin K, fresh frozen plasma or a prothrombin complex concentrate (PCC), such as beriplex or octaplex. PCCs are a combination of factors II, VII, IX and X with protein C and protein S, all of which are harvested from blood.

USES
- Prophylaxis of DVT
- Prevention of clot propagation in DVT/PE/vessel occlusion
- To prevent clot formation on extra-corporeal membranes, e.g. cardiopulmonary bypass circuits/haemofilters

MOA
- Binds to antithrombin III (ATIII) reversibly, and increases the rate at which ATIII binds to thrombin by 1000x
- Once thrombin is complexed with ATIII, clot formation is inhibited
- At low doses factor Xa inhibited
- At higher dose factors IXa, XIa, XIIa are inhibited
- At very high dose platelet aggregation is inhibited

EFFECTS
HAEMATOLOGICAL
- ↑ APTT
- ↑ TT
- ↑ ACT
- No effect on bleeding time
- Thrombocytopenia (type I). Non-immune, not usually significant. Platelet count recovers quickly on stopping drug
- Heparin-induced thrombocytopenia (Type II = 'HIT'). Immune mediated – heparin binds to platelets and complex removed by IgG

OTHER
- Osteoporosis
- Reverse with protamine
- Low molecular weight heparin works by inhibiting factor Xa via ATIII. Only needs once daily dosing, does not require monitoring

ABSORPTION/ DISTRIBUTION
- Not given orally
- $t_{1/2}$ 40–120 min
- Highly protein bound
- V_D 0.04–0.1 L/kg
- Low lipid solubility, so does not cross BBB or placenta
- $t_{1/2}$ 40–120 min

HEPARIN
(Unfractionated: 3000–40 000 Da)
Glycosaminoglycan
- Clear colourless solution
- Variable dose and potency depending on preparation

METABOLISM AND EXCRETION
- Metabolised in liver, kidney and reticuloendothelial system
- Excreted in urine

CHEMICAL PROPERTIES
- Nil

Warfarin

USES
- Prophylaxis of DVT/PE
- Prophylaxis of clot formation on prosthetic heart valves/in AF
- Prevention of clot propagation in DVT/PE/vessel occlusion

MOA
- Inhibits synthesis of vitamin K dependent clotting factors: II, VII, IX, X

Reduced Vit K   Oxidised Vit K

NAD+   NADH

Warfarin stops this

- Precursors of clotting factors synthesised in liver. They are then carboxylated and during this reaction Vit K is oxidised
- Warfarin prevents Vit K returning to its reduced state
- Only affects synthesis of new factors, takes 72 hours to work
- Action irreversible

ABSORPTION/ DISTRIBUTION
- Well absorbed orally
- Protein binding 99%
- V_D 0.1–0.16 L/kg
- $t_{1/2}$ 35–45 hours

EFFECTS
HAEMATOLOGICAL
- ↑ PT
- ↑ INR

DRUG INTERACTIONS
- Availability affected by drugs which induce/inhibit liver enzymes
- Cholestyramine decreases absorption of fat soluble vitamins A, D, E, and K therefore potentiates effect of warfarin

OTHER
- Hypersensitivity reactions
- Teratogenic in first trimester
- Crosses placenta and can cause fetal haemorrhage

PRE-OP
- Stop warfarin 1 week before elective surgery– replace with heparin if necessary. INR should be < 2 to operate
- Rapid reversal: beryplex/FFP
- Slow reversal (12 hours): Vit K

WARFARIN
Coumarin derivative
- Tablets: 0.5/1/3/5 mg

DOSE
- Patient-specific, titrate to effect
- Usually 2–9 mg/day

METABOLISM AND EXCRETION
- Hepatic metabolism
- Excreted in urine and faeces

CHEMICAL PROPERTIES
- Nil

31. ANTI-PLATELET AGENTS

Draw a diagram of a platelet showing all the receptors that are activated during platelet aggregation and adhesion.

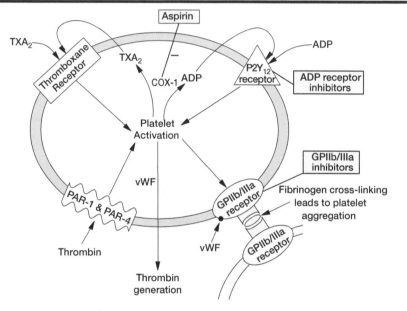

Fig. 31.1 Platelet showing main receptors involved in clot formation

> Membrane glycoproteins GPIa/IIa, GPVI and GPIV, function as receptors in platelet adhesion to collagen.
> GPIIb/IIIa (also known as integrin $\alpha_{IIb}\beta_3$) is a receptor for fibrinogen and von Willebrand factor.
> Adenosine diphosphate (ADP) binds to $P2Y_1$ (G_q) and $P2Y_{12}$ (G_i) receptors.
> Thrombin binds to protease-activated receptors (PARs), PAR-1 and PAR-4.
> Thromboxane A_2 (TxA_2) is produced from arachidonic acid through conversion by cyclo-oxygenase-1. The TxA_2 receptor (TP) is also activated by the prostaglandin endoperoxides PGG_2 and PGH_2.

How are platelets involved in clotting?

Platelets are critical in haemostasis and the development of arterial thrombi. Damaged endothelium initiates a multistep interaction between platelets and the adhesive macromolecules within the extracellular matrix, resulting in platelet activation, adhesion to the endothelium and platelet aggregation.

> **Initial contact:** von Willebrand factor (vWF) binds to GPIbα, and collagen bind to collagen receptor GPVI, activating platelets.
> **Platelet adhesion:** bound vWF activates GPIIb/IIIa membrane glycoproteins, allowing them to bind fibrinogen, resulting in a firm adhesion of platelets to the endothelium.
> **Platelet activation:** activated platelets release TxA$_2$ and ADP, which results in recruitment, activation and degranulation of surrounding platelets. Thrombin, a product of the coagulation cascade, also mediates this process. All three act via G-protein-coupled receptors (GPCRs), causing a conformational change in GPIIb/IIIa receptors.
> **Platelet aggregation:** fibrinogen binds to GPIIb/IIIa receptors, converts to fibrin and stabilises the thrombus by cross-linkage of platelets.

Platelet activation, adhesion and aggregation are inhibited by the endothelium-derived mediator nitric oxide (NO), also known as endothelium-derived relaxing factor (EDRF), and prostacyclin (PGI$_2$). These mediators act via GPCRs, increasing intracellular levels of cyclic adenosine monophosphate (cAMP) and cyclic guanosine monophosphate (cGMP) in platelets, thereby inhibiting them.

How can anti-platelet agents be classified?

> Anti-platelet agents decrease platelet aggregation and inhibit thrombus formation.
> They are most effective in the treatment or prevention of arterial clots that are composed largely of platelets, where anticoagulants have little effect.
> The main anti-platelet agents in clinical use are:
>   • Cyclo-oxygenase (COX) inhibitors
>   • ADP receptor inhibitors (thienopyridines and non-thienopyridines)
>   • Dipyridamole
>   • Parenteral GPIIb/IIIa inhibitors
>   • Other agents include thromboxane inhibitors and PAR-1 antagonists.

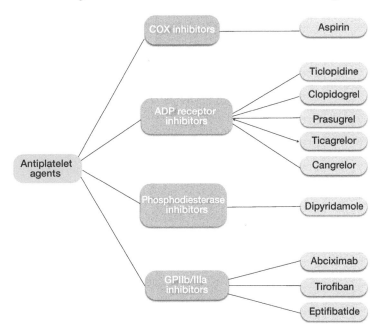

Fig. 31.2   Classification of anti-platelet agents

What are the mechanisms of action of anti-platelet agents?

Aspirin:
> Changes the balance between prostacyclin (which inhibits platelet aggregation) and thromboxane (which promotes aggregation).
> It irreversibly and non-selectively acetylates and inhibits the enzyme COX, and is 50–100 times more effective against COX-1.
> The conversion of arachidonic acid (AA) to endoperoxide (EPO) is inhibited with resultant prevention of synthesis of TxA_2 in platelets and prostacyclin (PGI_2) in endothelial cells.
> The vascular endothelium recovers and can synthesise more prostacyclin, but thromboxane synthesis only recovers after new platelets are formed.

ADP receptor blockers
> Thienopyridines (e.g. ticlopidine, clopidogrel and prasugrel)
  • Act by inhibiting the ADP-dependent pathway of platelet activation.
  • They are prodrugs whose active metabolites inhibit the $P2Y_{12}$ subtype of the ADP receptor, preventing binding of adenosine diphosphate (ADP) to its receptor on the platelet surface.
  • They are competitive antagonists and their effects are irreversible.
  • Platelet function returns to normal with the formation of new platelets in 7–10 days.
> Ticagrelor
  • New drug that indirectly inhibits ADP.
  • It acts on an independent ligand-binding site on the $P2Y_{12}$ receptor, which results in a conformational change in the receptor, rendering it inactive.
  • This process displays dose-dependent, reversible non-competitive binding with ADP.
> Cangrelor
  • New, rapidly acting, reversible ADP blocker that binds selectively and specifically to the $P2Y_{12}$ receptor on the platelet surface.
  • It has a rapid onset and offset of action, and does not require activation or conversion by the liver to an active metabolite.
  • It is administered by i.v. infusion, with a plasma half-life of 3–5 minutes, resulting in full recovery of platelet activity within 60 minutes.

Dipyridamole
> Inhibits cellular uptake of adenosine by platelets, erythrocytes and endothelial cells, increasing the extracellular concentration of adenosine, which increases cAMP levels within the platelets.
> Also inhibits platelet phosphodiesterases (PDEs), which normally break down cAMP and cGMP to inactive molecules.
> Elevated levels of cAMP and cGMP inhibit activation and aggregation of platelets (by blocking the platelet response to ADP).
> In high doses, it is also a potent vasodilator.

GPIIb/IIIa inhibitors (e.g. abciximab and tirofiban)
> Have the greatest antiplatelet activity as they inhibit the final common pathway of platelet aggregation where fibrinogen binds to the GPIIb/IIIa receptor.
> Platelet inhibition is reversible with return of normal platelet function by 48 hours with abciximab and by 6–8 hours with tirofiban.
> They are administered parenterally and are primarily used in the management of acute coronary syndromes (ACS) and percutaneous coronary interventions (PCI).

What are the peri-operative considerations for anti-platelet agents (i.e. when to stop for surgery and neuroaxial blocks)?

With increasing use of anti-platelet agents in an ageing population, much consideration has been given to peri-operative management. Each patient should be stratified according to individual thrombotic and surgical bleeding risk and joint multidisciplinary team involvement in the decision-making process (surgeon, anaesthetist, cardiologist, haematologist) is recommended.

Aspirin monotherapy:
> Primary prevention or AF: can be safely discontinued 7–10 days before surgery.
> Secondary prevention with low risk of bleeding: relative risk is in favour of continuation.
> High risk of bleeding (cardiac, intracranial, prostate and hip surgery): discontinue 7–10 days before surgery.

Dual anti-platelet therapy (aspirin & ADP inhibitors):
> Low-risk situations: ADP inhibitors should be discontinued 5–7 days before surgery, and aspirin should be continued.
> High-cardiovascular risk (recent MI, PCI, BMS <6 weeks, DES <12 months, risk of myocardial ischaemia/infarct):
  • Delay elective surgery
  • Proceed with emergency surgery despite no discontinuation in DAPT. May require platelet transfusion in life-threatening bleeding.
  • Urgent surgery where bleeding risk is high: may require complete discontinuation of anti-platelet medications. In these situations, bridging therapies, such as heparin or GPIIb/IIIa inhibitors, should be considered

Regional anaesthesia:
> Carries a relative risk of bleeding in patients on anti-platelet agents.
> Guidelines published by the Association of Anaesthetists of Great Britain and Ireland in 2013 recommend risk should be minimised by:
  • Ensuring that neuraxial and peripheral nerve blocks are performed by experienced clinicians
  • Where possible they should be performed under ultrasound guidance
  • Stopping anti-platelet agents where applicable in a timely manner.
> Procedures carrying the greatest risk of haematoma are epidural with a catheter, one-shot epidural, spinal, paravertebral blocks, deep blocks, and superficial perivascular blocks. Fascial blocks, superficial blocks and local infiltration approach normal risk.

Table 31.1 Timeframes for stopping anti-platelet therapy

Drug	Time after stopping drug before block performance	Administration of drug while spinal or epidural catheter in place	Time to next drug dose after block performance or catheter removal
NSAIDs or aspirin	No additional precautions	No additional precautions	No additional precautions
Clopidogrel	7 days	Not recommended	6 hours
Prasugrel	7 days	Not recommended	6 hours
Ticagrelor	5 days	Not recommended	6 hours
Tirofiban	8 hours	Not recommended	6 hours
Abciximab	48 hours	Not recommended	6 hours
Dipyridamole	No additional precautions	No additional precautions	6 hours

32. BLOOD

Blood transfusion may be life-saving, but it is not without risk. Many issues may be covered in an examination question including composition and storage of blood, risks and benefits of transfusion, effects of massive blood transfusion, infective and immunological effects of blood transfusion, and blood conservation strategies.

Describe the composition and storage of blood.

Whole blood is separated into red cells, plasma and platelets via centrifugation. Once separated plasma must be frozen as soon as possible to under −18 °C, red cells must be stored at 1–6 °C and platelets must be stored at room temperature (20–24 °C) on shaking platforms (lifespan 3–5 days).

Leucodepletion is then performed in order to remove the white blood cells via filtration. Leucodeplete blood minimises the chances of alloimmunisation, reduces the incidence of febrile transfusion reactions and reduces the chances of cytomegalovirus (CMV) transmission.

Severely immunosuppressed patients require irradiated blood in order to prevent donor T-lymphocytes dividing in the recipient, which can result in transfusion and associated graft-versus-host disease. Stem cell transplant (immunosuppressed) patients will also require CMV-negative blood. The following changes occur in stored blood:

> Fall in 2,3 DPG levels
> Left shift of the oxyhaemoglobin dissociation curve
> Fall in pH (to approximately 7.0)
> Rise in potassium concentration

Storage solutions include:
> **Acid-citrate-dextrose:** Citrate acts as an anticoagulant by binding calcium while dextrose is an energy source for glycolysis. Red cell survival is 21 days.
> **Citrate-phosphate-dextrose:** Increases red cell survival to 28 days.
> **Citrate-phosphate-dextrose-adenine:** The addition of adenine increases red cell ATP thereby increasing red cell survival to 35 days.
> **Saline (140 mmol/L)-adenine (1.5 mmol/L)-glucose (50 mmol/L)-mannitol (30 mmol/L):** Allows a greater volume of plasma to be removed from blood in order to use plasma for coagulation factors.

Discuss the risks and benefits of transfusion.

The principal benefit of red cell transfusion is the improvement in oxygen-carrying capacity by increasing haemoglobin levels. Raising the haematocrit has also been shown to improve microcirculation in trauma and septic patients.

However, there are multiple risks and complications:

> **Haemolytic transfusion reaction**, e.g. life-threatening ABO incompatibility versus delayed haemolysis to minor red cell antigens
> **Febrile reactions**
> **Infection transmission:** HIV (1 in 4 000 000), hepatitis A, hepatitis B, hepatitis C, malaria, variant CJD, CMV, syphilis, HTLV
> **Metabolic:** hyperkalaemia and hypocalcaemia
> **Hypothermia:** transfusion of cold stored blood
> **Circulatory overload:** cardiac failure
> **Immune:** graft-versus-host disease and possible increase in colorectal tumour recurrence rates
> **Transfusion-related acute lung injury (TRALI):** incidence has fallen since the introduction of leucocyte-deplete blood
> **Iron overload** in chronic transfusion
> **Septic shock** from bacterial contamination of donor blood
> **Impaired coagulation:** If red cells are transfused rapidly in large volumes the liver's ability to clear the citrate may be overwhelmed and coagulation may become impaired.

What constitutes a massive transfusion?

> There are many different definitions of what constitutes a massive transfusion, but they all define a volume of transfusion and a time period, e.g. 10 units of blood within 6 hours or replacement of entire circulating volume with transfused blood within 24 hours.
> The aim of treatment is the rapid and effective restoration of an adequate blood volume to maintain blood composition within safe limits with regards to haemostasis, oxygen-carrying capacity, oncotic pressure and biochemistry.

What are the problems encountered during massive transfusion?

Massive blood transfusion encompasses all of the risks of individual blood unit transfusion listed above but also has other specific problems:

> **Thrombocytopenia:** Dilutional thrombocytopenia is inevitable following massive transfusion as platelet function declines to zero after only a few days of storage. It has been shown that at least 1.5 times blood volume must be replaced for this to become a clinical problem. However, thrombocytopenia can occur following smaller transfusions if disseminated intravascular coagulation (DIC) occurs or there is pre-existing thrombocytopenia.
> **Coagulation factor depletion:** Stored blood contains all coagulation factors except V and VIII. Production of these factors is increased by the stress response to trauma. Therefore, only mild changes in coagulation are due to the transfusion per se, and supervening DIC is more likely to be responsible for disordered haemostasis. DIC is a consequence of delayed or inadequate resuscitation, and the usual explanation for abnormal coagulation indices out of proportion to the volume of blood transfused.

> **Oxygen affinity changes:** Massive transfusion of stored blood with high oxygen affinity adversely affects oxygen delivery to the tissues. However, 2,3 DPG levels rise rapidly following transfusion and normal oxygen affinity is usually restored in a few hours.

> **Hypocalcaemia:** Each unit of blood contains approximately 3 g citrate, which binds ionised calcium. The healthy adult liver will metabolise 3 g citrate every 5 minutes. Transfusion at rates higher than one unit every 5 minutes or impaired liver function may thus lead to citrate toxicity and hypocalcaemia.

> **Hyperkalaemia:** The plasma potassium concentration of stored blood increases during storage and may be over 30 mmol/L. Hyperkalaemia is generally not a problem unless very large amounts of blood are given quickly. On the contrary, hypokalaemia is more common as red cells begin active metabolism and intracellular uptake of potassium restarts.

> **Acid–base disturbances:** Lactic acid levels in the blood pack give stored blood an acid load of up to 30–40 mmol/L. This, along with citric acid, is usually metabolised rapidly. Indeed, citrate is metabolised to bicarbonate, and a profound metabolic alkalosis may ensue.
> The acid–base status of the recipient is usually of more importance, final acid–base status being dependent on tissue perfusion, rate of administration and citrate metabolism.

> **Hypothermia:** Leads to reduction in citrate and lactate metabolism (leading to hypocalcaemia and metabolic acidosis), increase in affinity of haemoglobin for oxygen, impairment of red cell deformability, platelet dysfunction and an increased tendency to cardiac dysrhythmias.

> **Acute respiratory distress syndrome (ARDS):** The aetiology of ARDS is as yet not fully understood, but various risk factors have been identified. Both under– and over-transfusion are associated with an increased risk of ARDS, as is albumin <30 g/L. Microaggregate filters should be used during massive transfusion except when giving fresh whole blood or platelets.

During massive blood transfusion, specific component therapy is required, namely FFP 12 mL/kg, to provide coagulation factors, platelets (keep count >50 000), cryoprecipitate for fibrinogen replacement (if fibrinogen <1.0 g/L).

In major haemorrhage blood products are generally given in a 1:1:1 ratio. That is one unit packed red cells:one unit of FFP :one unit of platelets. It should be noted that one pool of platelets is made up of the platelets taken from five donated units of blood. Hence, platelets should be given after every 10 units of blood products (i.e. five units red cells + five units FFP + one pool platelets). Calcium levels are checked after every 10 units and levels should be kept in the normal range.

If blood products are given in the ratios above and patients are kept warm coagulation normally remains effective. In some cases of major haemorrhage recombinant factor (rF) VII may be required to boost coagulation.

What blood conservation strategies are available?

Remembering that blood transfusion can be associated with morbidity and mortality, there exist a number of strategies with the aim of reducing the need for transfusion.

> **Restrictive red cell transfusion trigger** – Accepting a lower haemoglobin level that is safe for the individual patient, e.g. 10 g/dL for a patient with ischaemic heart disease or as low as 7 g/dL for a fit 20-year old.

> **Pre-donation** – Patients for planned surgery with significant expected blood loss may be candidates for pre-donation of blood followed by intra-operative transfusion of their own blood.

> **Hypotensive anaesthesia** – Used in certain types of surgery such as middle ear surgery or neurosurgery to reduce blood loss.

> **Anti-fibrinolytic agents** – Tranexamic acid and aprotinin inhibit clot breakdown.

> **Intra-operative blood salvage via cell savers** – Used in certain types of surgery.

> **Recombinant factor VII** – Used in haemophilia and in massive bleeding, provided platelet count is adequate (not effective in the setting of thrombocytopenia).

> **Artificial oxygen carriers** – Perfluorocarbons and modified haemoglobins are the two main products. Oxygen transport characteristics of perfluorocarbon emulsions are fundamentally different from those of blood. Blood exhibits a sigmoidal oxygen dissociation curve. In contrast, perfluorocarbon emulsions are characterised by a linear relationship between oxygen partial pressure and oxygen content. Elevated arterial oxygen partial pressures are thus beneficial to maximise the oxygen transport capacity of perfluorocarbon emulsions. No artificial oxygen carriers are used extensively within the UK at present.

33. HYPOGLYCAEMIC AGENTS

What classes of drugs are used to treat type 1 diabetes mellitus (DM)?

> Insulin is the main class of drug used to treat type 1 DM.
> Insulin treatment has been available since 1925, initially extracted from beef and pork pancreases. In the 1980s this was replaced by synthetic human insulin, which is now largely being replaced by genetically engineered human insulin analogues. Human and animal insulins, when injected subcutaneously, are more likely to clump, resulting in a slower onset of action and longer, more unpredictable duration of action when compared to insulin analogues. They are, therefore, more likely to cause hypoglycaemia between meals and at night, followed by fasting hyperglycaemia.
> Insulins can be categorised according to onset of action, peak and duration of action.
> The main groups are rapid-, short-, intermediate- and long-acting (*see* table below).
> Biphasic insulins are ready mixed combinations of rapid- or short-acting insulins with intermediate-acting insulins.

Table 33.1 Types of insulins

Type of Insulin	Onset	Peak	Duration	Administration timing
Rapid-acting insulin analogues (aspart/Novorapid®, lyspro/ Humalog®, glulisine/Apidra®)	<15 min	1–2 h	4–6 h	Shortly before, during or immediately after meals
Short-acting human insulin (regular soluble: Actrapid®/ Humulin R®)	0.5–1 h	2–4 h	6–8 h	30 min before meals (also used for IV infusions)
Intermediate-acting human insulin (isophane/NPH/ Humulin I®, Insulatard®)	1–2 h	6–10 h	>12 h	Twice daily regimens (before morning and evening meals)
Long-acting insulin analogues (glargine/Lantus®, detemir/ Levemir®)	1–1.5 h	Flat, maximal effect in 5 h	12–24 h (detemir) 24 h (glargine)	Once or twice daily (physiologically similar to endogenous basal insulin secretion)

What different types of insulin treatment regimens are you aware of?

> **Once daily:** only suitable for type 2 diabetes.
> **Twice daily:** biphasic insulin is used. Episodes of hypoglycaemia followed by fasting hyperglycaemia may be minimised by using rapid-acting analogues instead of short-acting human insulins.

> **Basal-bolus:** intermediate- or long-acting insulin is used at bedtime, in combination with rapid- or short-acting insulin at mealtimes.
> **Continuous subcutaneous insulin infusion (CSII) or insulin pump therapy:** useful for type 1 diabetics with recurrent hypoglycaemia, pre-breakfast hyperglycaemia, poorly controlled glucose on multiple daily injections, unpredictable lives or delayed meals.

What classes of drugs are used to treat type 2 diabetes?

There are two main families of drugs that are used – oral hypoglycaemics and non-insulin injectables.

Oral hypoglycaemic agents:
These agents are either used singly or in combination. They can be classified as follows:

Biguanides
> Metformin is the only licensed drug in this group.
> MOA: it enhances uptake of glucose in skeletal muscle cells via the glucose transporter protein GLUT4, and can only act in the presence of endogenous insulin, therefore requiring pancreatic islet cells with residual function.
> Indication and benefits: first-line drug in overweight (and increasingly all) type 2 diabetics. It causes less hypoglycaemia and weight gain than sulphonylureas and reduces macrovascular complications, stroke and death. It may be of benefit in overweight type 1 diabetics.
> Side effects: lactic acidosis (especially in patients with renal insufficiency, liver disease, cardiovascular disease, peripheral vascular disease, pulmonary disease, and those aged over 65) and gastrointestinal (GI) side effects.
> Contraindication: renal failure (serum creatinine >150 µmol/L or eGFR <30 mL/min/1.73 m^2)

Insulin secretagogues:
> **Sulphonylureas**
  • Gliclazide, glipizide, glimipramide, glibenclamide, tolbutamide
  • MOA: they promote the secretion of insulin from pancreatic islet cells (they bind to ATP-dependent potassium channels on islet cell membranes, cause depolarisation and voltage-gated calcium channels to open, resulting in fusion of insulin granules with the cell membrane and release of pro-insulin). They also act on the liver to promote glycolysis and inhibit the production of glucose. Most have duration of action of 12–24 hours; tolbutamide is short-acting (half-life of 4.5–6.5 hours).
  • Indication and benefits: first-line drug in type 2 diabetes when metformin is contraindicated or not tolerated. They are effective at long-term reduction of glycosylated haemoglobin (HbA1c).
  • Side effects: hypoglycaemia (especially in patients with renal and hepatic impairment and in the elderly), weight gain, liver dysfunction and GI disturbance.

> **Meglitinides**
  • Repaglinide and nateglinide are the only two licensed for use in the UK.
  • MOA: they are rapid-acting stimulators of insulin secretion and are taken before meals. They act by binding to various sites on pancreatic beta cells.
  • Indications: used in combination with metformin where sulphonylureas are not tolerated, and especially in patients with erratic eating habits. Repaglinide can also be used as monotherapy in non-obese patients where metformin is contraindicated or not tolerated.
  • Side effects: hypoglycaemia.

> **Thiazolidinediones (TDZ or 'glitazones')**
  • Pioglitazone is the only one currently licensed for use in the UK.
  • MOA: increases hepatic sensitivity to insulin, promoting glucose clearance, and is particularly effective in patients with insulin resistance.
  • Indications: used in combination with either metformin or a sulphonylurea where one or the other is not tolerated or is contraindicated. Also used as monotherapy or in combination with insulin.
  • Side effects: increased risks of heart failure due to fluid retention (rosiglitazone was withdrawn in 2010 for this reason and for its increased risk of MI), hepatic enzyme derangement and liver failure (rare), limb fractures (in women with other risk factors for fractures) and bladder cancer.
  • Contraindications: congestive cardiac failure, patients at increased risk of fractures.

> **Alpha glucosidase inhibitors (acarbose)**
  • MOA: inhibition of intestinal alpha glucosidase, resulting in delayed absorption and digestion of sucrose and starch.
  • Indications: in combination with metformin or sulphonylureas, or as monotherapy where other hypoglycaemic agents are not tolerated or contraindicated.
  • Side effects: high chance of GI adverse effects, particularly flatulence and diarrhoea.

> **Dipeptidyl peptidase-4 (DPP-4) inhibitors**
  • Sitagliptin and vildagliptin
  • MOA: DPP-4 inhibitors ultimately increase insulin secretion and lower glucagon secretion. Inhibition of the enzyme DPP-4 results in reduced breakdown and increased levels of incretins, which are GI hormones including glucagon-like peptide-1 (GLP-1) and gastric inhibitory peptide (GIP). Incretins increase insulin release from beta cells and delay absorption of nutrients by reducing gastric emptying.
  • Indications: used in combination with metformin, sulphonylureas, or TDZ. Can also be used as monotherapy. Sitagliptin may also be added to insulin treatment.
  • Side effects: hypersensitivity reactions: anaphylaxis, angioedema and Stevens–Johnson syndrome.

Non-insulin injectables:
Glucagon-like peptide-1 mimetics (exenatide)
  > MOA: acts as incretin-mimetic and is given by twice-daily subcutaneous injection before meals.
  > Indications: in combination with metformin or sulphonylureas, or as an alternative to insulin in obese patients on maximal doses of oral treatments.
  > Side effects: significant weight loss (therefore appropriate for patients with BMI >35 kg.m^2).

What are the NICE guidelines on the management of type 2 DM?

The recommendations by NICE were initially published in 2009 and updated in 2014. The management of type 2 DM is complex, requires blood glucose and HbA1c monitoring, and caters for individual indications, contraindications, lifestyles and circumstances. In its entirety the guideline is beyond the scope of the FRCA exams, however, a brief description is as follows:

> **First-line treatment:**
>   • Metformin in overweight (and in non-overweight) patients.
>   • Sulphonylurea where patient is not overweight or cannot have metformin.
>   • Rapid-acting secretagogue (meglitinides) in people with erratic lifestyles.
>   • Acarbose where the above are not tolerated/contraindicated.
> **Second-line treatment:**
>   • Sulphonylurea to first-line metformin.
>   • Metformin to first-line sulphonylurea.
>   • Meglitinides to first-line metformin.
>   • DPP-4 inhibitors or TDZ to first-line metformin or sulphonylurea.
> **Third-line treatment**
>   • Insulin to metformin and sulphonylurea.
>   • Exenatide to metformin and sulphonylurea.
>   • DPP-4 inhibitor or TDZ to metformin and sulphonylurea.

DPP-4 inhibitors, TDZ and GLP-1 mimetics should only be continued beyond 6 months if there has been a beneficial metabolic response (HbA1c decrease).

34. ANTICONVULSANTS

What is epilepsy and how is it classified?

Epilepsy is a chronic disease resulting from paroxysmal, episodic, abnormal and spontaneous discharge of electrical activity in the brain. It can be classified as follows:

Fig. 34.1 Classification of epilepsy

Which drugs are available to treat epilepsy and how do they work?

There are a wide variety of anticonvulsants available, but their mechanisms of action can be divided into two main groups:

> **Drugs enhancing GABA-mediated inhibition** – benzodiazepines, barbiturates, sodium valproate and vigabatrin.
> **Drugs modulating sodium flux in nerves** – phenytoin and carbamazepine.

This latter group of drugs exert their effect by binding to inactivated fast Na^+ channels, reducing the flux of Na^+ into cells and stabilising their membranes. Ca^{2+} and K^+ efflux are also reduced. Their anticonvulsant effect is probably achieved by preventing the repetitive opening and closing of fast Na^+ channels, so that the sodium current is reduced until it no longer provokes an action potential.

Drugs enhancing GABA-mediated inhibition:
> **Benzodiazepines,** e.g. diazepam (see spider diagrams, Chapter 37, 'Miscellaneous drugs', benzodiazepines).
Benzodiazepines (BDZ) appear to have their own specific receptors, which are closely coupled to the GABA$_A$ receptor. When a BDZ binds it facilitates the binding of GABA to its respective receptor. BDZs exert their effect by increasing the frequency of opening of the GABA$_A$ channels. There are two types of BDZ receptor:
  - **BDZ1** found in the spinal cord and cerebellum. Stimulation causes anxiolysis.
  - **BDZ2** found in the spinal cord, hippocampus and cerebral cortex. Stimulation causes sedation and has an anticonvulsant effect.

> **Barbiturates**, e.g. phenobarbitone
Barbiturates increase the duration of opening of the GABA$_A$ chloride channel when stimulated.

> **Sodium valproate** – refer to the spider diagram
> **Vigabatrin:** This reversibly inhibits GABA transaminase, the enzyme that breaks down GABA.

Drugs modulating sodium flux in nerves:
> **Phenytoin** – refer to spider diagram
> **Carbamazepine** – refer to the spider diagram

How would you anaesthetise a patient with epilepsy?

Pre-operative assessment: Take a full and through anaesthetic history, paying close attention to the following:
> History of the epileptic activity
> Underlying pathology or lesion causing the seizures
> Type, frequency and duration of the seizures and when the last one occurred
> Occupation and driving status
> Drug history. It is important that the patient receives their medication in a timely manner. If they are nil by mouth for any prolonged period, appropriate medication should be given by an alternative route, e.g. rectally or intravenously. This should be discussed with a neurologist.

Pre-operative care:
> Induce anaesthesia using thiopentone.
> Avoid ketamine and etomidate as they can lower the seizure threshold.
> Anticonvulsants induce liver enzyme activity and therefore the patient may need increased doses of anaesthetic agents and muscle relaxants.
> Avoid hypoxia and hypercapnia throughout the procedure as these states can lower the seizure threshold.
> Avoid tramadol as this can lower seizure thresholds.

Propofol is said to cause epileptiform movements, but it has not been shown to produce epileptiform activity on the EEG. In some units it is used in the treatment of status epilepticus and so it is probably safe for routine use in patients with epilepsy.

Describe the GABA receptor.

GABA (gamma amino-butyric acid) is the main inhibitory neurotransmitter in the CNS. The activation of the GABA receptor causes increased flux of chloride or potassium ions into the cell and causes hyperpolarisation of the membrane, therefore stabilising the synapse. There are two GABA receptor subtypes:

> **GABA$_A$:** A ligand-gated chloride ion channel, with five receptor subunits (2α, 2β, γ) arranged around the ion channel. These are found on the post-synaptic membrane.
> **GABA$_B$:** A G-protein-coupled receptor. Stimulation of GABA$_B$ causes increased potassium conductance. These are found on both the pre- and postsynaptic membranes. Baclofen acts via these receptors.

Phenytoin

USES
- Treatment and prophylaxis of tonic-clonic seizures
- Trigeminal neuralgia
- Antiarrhythmic (Class 1b) used to treat ventricular arrhythmias of tricyclic and digoxin overdose

MOA
- Binds to inactivated fast Na^+ channels reducing flux of Na^+ into cells and stabilising the membrane
- Ca^{2+} and K^+ efflux also reduced
- Anticonvulsant effect probably achieved by preventing repetitive opening and closing of fast Na^+ channels, so that the sodium current is reduced until it no longer provokes an action potential

EFFECTS
CVS
- Class 1b shortens refractory period of cardiac muscle. Rapid injection can cause heart block, VF and asystole
CNS
- Antiepileptic
SIDE-EFFECTS
Idiosyncratic:
- Hirsuitism
- Coarse facies
- Acne
- Gum hyperplasia
- Megaloblastic anaemia
- Aplastic anaemia
- Rashes
- SLE
- Peripheral neuropathy
Concentration-dependent:
- Nausea and vomiting
- Tremor
- Ataxia
- Nystagmus
- Vertigo
- Drowsiness
Teratogenicity:
- Craniofacial abnormalities
- Limb abnormalities
- Cardiac abnormalities
- Growth retardation

ABSORPTION/ DISTRIBUTION
- Oral bioavailability 90%
- Protein binding 90%
- V_D 0.5 L/kg

METABOLISM AND EXCRETION
- Hepatic metabolism
- Exhibits zero order kinetics just above therapeutic range so care should be taken with dosing so as not to cause toxicity
- 80% renally excreted
- Potent liver enzyme inducer, so check for drug interactions
- Increases the required dose of aminosteroid muscle relaxants by 80%
- May decrease MAC of volatiles

PHENYTOIN
Anticonvulsant
Class 1b antiarrhythmic
- Capsules: 25/50/100/300 mg
- Syrup: 6 mg/mL
- Solution: 50 mg/mL

DOSE
- Loading: 15 mg/kg for treatment of seizure
- Maintenance: 100 mg 8 hourly
- Oral dose: 200–600 mg daily
- Therapeutic range: 10–20 mg/L

CHEMICAL PROPERTIES
- Nil

Sodium valproate

USES
- Treatment of epilepsy, especially generalised seizures and infantile spasms
- Chronic pain
- Mood stabiliser in mental illness

MOA
- Inhibits succinic semialdehyde dehydrogenase and so increases brain levels of GABA
- It may have some stabilising effect on sodium channels
- May mimic the action of GABA at postsynaptic receptors

ABSORPTION/ DISTRIBUTION
- Oral bioavailability almost 100%
- Protein binding 90%
- V_D 0.1–0.4 L/kg
- $t_{1/2}$ 8–20 hours

EFFECTS
CNS
- Antiepileptic
- Drowsiness
GI
- Hepatic dysfunction (contraindicated in liver disease. Monitor LFTs with chronic use)
- Pancreatitis
- Nausea and vomiting
OTHER
- Hair loss
- Weight gain
- Oedema
HAEMATOLOGICAL
- Thrombocytopenia and ↓ aggregation (check platelet function prior to regional/neuroaxial blockade)
- Impaired clotting reported

METABOLISM AND EXCRETION
- Hepatic metabolism
- Small amout excreted in urine, unchanged

SODIUM VALPROATE
Anticonvulsant
- Tablets: 100/200/500 mg
- Syrup: 40 mg/mL
- Powder: 400 mg ampoules for dissolution in water

DOSE
- 600–2500 mg/day in 2 divided doses
- Therapeutic range 40–100 mg/L

CHEMICAL PROPERTIES
- Nil

Carbamazepine

USES
- Treatment of epilepsy, especially generalised seizures and infantile spasms
- Chronic pain
- Mood stabiliser in mental illness

MOA
- Binds to inactivated fast Na^+ channels reducing flux of Na^+ into cells and stabilising the membrane
- Ca^{2+} and K^+ efflux also reduced
- Anticonvulsant effect probably achieved by preventing repetitive opening and closing of fast Na^+ channels, so that the sodium current is reduced until it no longer provokes an action potential

EFFECTS
CVS
- Depresses AV conduction and antiarrhythmic
CNS
- Antiepileptic
- Headache
- Diplopia
- Ataxia
- Sedation
GI
- Nausea and vomiting
- Hepatitis – monitor LFTs
HAEMATOLOGY
- Agranulocytosis
- Mild neutropenia
- Aplastic anaemia
OTHER
- Teratogenic
- Rashes
- Increases required dose of aminosteroid muscle relaxants by 80%
- Must monitor LFTs with chronic use

ABSORPTION/ DISTRIBUTION
- Almost 100% oral bioavailability
- Protein binding 75%
- V_D 1 L/kg
- $t_{1/2}$ 16–36 hours

CARBAMAZEPINE
Anticonvulsant
- Tablets: 100/200/400 mg
- Suppositories: 125/250 mg
- Syrup: 20 mg/mL white

DOSE
- 100–1600 mg/day

METABOLISM AND EXCRETION
- Hepatic metabolism to active compound
- With chronic use, induces liver enzymes and enhances own metabolism
- Excreted in urine

CHEMICAL PROPERTIES
- Nil

35. ANTIDEPRESSANTS

Depression is thought to occur, due to an imbalance in neurotransmitters such as serotonin, norepinephrine and dopamine. Antidepressants work by altering the balance of these central neurotransmitters.

The different classes of antidepressants differ in the neurotransmitters they affect. This determines their side effect profile and potential drug interactions.

All antidepressant drugs are prone to causing dependence syndromes, particularly drug withdrawal, and pre-operative discontinuation should be avoided or be gradual in the case of monoamine oxidase inhibitors.

Antidepressants are used to treat many other conditions such as anxiety disorders, obsessive-compulsive disorders, eating disorders, post-traumatic stress disorder, attention-deficit and hyperactivity disorders.

What are the different classes of antidepressant agents? Describe their mode of action, side effects and anaesthetic implications.

Monoamine oxidase inhibitors (MAOIs)
First class of antidepressant to be developed. Used infrequently now due to potentially lethal interactions with drugs and tyramine-containing foods.

Mode of action:
> Prevents breakdown of monoamine neurotransmitters by inhibiting monoamine oxidase (MAO) enzyme.
> MAOs exist in two isoforms:
  • MAO-A (selectively breaks down serotonin, epinephrine and norepinephrine)
  • MAO-B (selectively breaks down phenethylamine)
  • Both break down dopamine.
> Older agents inhibit both MAO-A and MAO-B.
> Newer agents (e.g. moclobemide) selectively inhibit MAO-A and are classed as RIMAs (reversible inhibitors of monoamine oxidase-A).
> MAO-B inhibitors (e.g. selegiline) are used as anti-Parkinson's medications due to their dopaminergic properties.

Side effects:
> Hypertension and hypertensive crises – both types of MAOs breakdown tyramine (a chemical present in aged cheese and wines). MAOIs decrease tyramine breakdown, leading to increased plasma concentrations, which can elevate blood pressure.
> Serotonin syndrome when used with other serotonergic agents.
> Orthostatic hypotension.
> Psychosis, headaches, insomnia, sexual dysfunction, weight gain.

Implications for anaesthesia:
> Treatment should be gradually discontinued pre-operatively. If treatment continued (e.g. emergency case) a benzodiazepine premedication should be used.
> MAOIs reduce metabolism of barbiturates, so lower doses should be used. Avoid ketamine. Propofol, etomidate, benzodiazepines, inhalation agents can all be used safely.

> Morphine, fentanyl, alfentanil and remifentanil can all be used safely.
> Avoid tramadol, pethidine and linezolid as they can precipitate serotonin syndrome.
> Avoid pancuronium as it can cause noradrenaline release.
> Local anaesthetics containing adrenaline should be used with caution.
> Indirect-acting sympathomimetics (e.g. ephedrine) are absolutely contraindicated as they may precipitate potentially fatal hypertensive crises.
> Direct-acting sympathomimetics (e.g. phenylephrine) should be administered at lower doses.

Tricyclic antidepressants

Named for their chemical structure containing three rings. They have now largely been replaced by second-generation antidepressants with a more favourable side effect profile. They are also used to treat chronic and neuropathic pain. Examples include imipramine, amitriptyline, doxepin and dosulepin.

Mode of action:
> Act primarily as serotonin–norepinephrine re-uptake inhibitors by blocking the serotonin transporter (SERT) and norepinephrine transporter (NET) on the presynaptic membrane, resulting in a higher concentration of neurotransmitters in the synaptic cleft, and increased neurotransmission.
> Also act as antagonists at multiple other receptor sites including 5-HT, α_1.adrenergic, NMDA, H_1 and H_2, and mACh receptors. These additional actions contribute to their efficacy as antidepressants and to their side effect profile.
> Many are potent inhibitors of sodium channels and L-type calcium channels (they act like class 1 anti-arrhythmic agents). This effect is potentially cardiotoxic and is responsible for the high risk of mortality when taken in overdose.

Side effects:
> Anticholinergic effects – dry mouth, dry nose, blurred vision, constipation, urinary retention, sweating and increased body temperature.
> Changes in appetite and weight, nausea and vomiting, sexual dysfunction.
> CNS – drowsiness, confusion, muscle twitches. In overdose – seizures, hallucinations, hyper-reflexia, myoclonus and coma.
> CVS – postural hypotension, tachycardia, arrhythmias. In overdose – hypotension or transient hypertension, ventricular tachyarrhythmias (VT and VF) and ECG changes (sinus tachycardia, prolonged QRS, QT and PR intervals).

Implications for anaesthesia:
> Continue peri-operatively.
> Increased levels of central neurotransmitters may increase anaesthetic requirement.
> Depleted levels of cardiac catecholamines may potentiate cardiac depressant effects of anaesthesia.
> Increased response to anticholinergics. Atropine, which crosses the blood–brain barrier, may lead to post-operative confusion.
> Exaggerated BP response to indirect-acting sympathomimetics, which should be avoided, and direct-acting sympathomimetics, which should be used in lower doses.
> Avoid ketamine, pancuronium, epinephrine-containing solutions and sympathetic stimulation.

Overdose:
> TCAs have a narrow therapeutic index and are readily absorbed in the alkaline environment of the small intestine; therefore severe symptoms may occur within 1 hour of overdose.
> Symptoms include anticholinergic effects, cardio- and neurotoxicity as described above, pulmonary hypoventilation due to CNS depression and reduced gut motility with absent bowel sounds. Metabolic and respiratory acidosis can occur.
> Treatment includes both supportive and specific measures:
  • ITU monitoring for symptomatic patients with continuous BP, ECG, and frequent CNS and arterial pH monitoring, with ventilatory support if required.
  • Activated charcoal to adsorb TCA in stomach (if within 2 hours of ingestion), although other methods of gastric decontamination are not recommended.
  • Maintain normothermia
  • IV sodium bicarbonate infusion and fluids in the presence of metabolic acidosis (TCAs are highly protein bound and become less bound in acidic environments. By reversing the acidosis, protein binding increases and bioavailability is reduced). The sodium load may help to reverse sodium channel blockade.
  • Antiarrhythmics such as phenytoin and magnesium may be required if dysrhythmia is refractory to sodium bicarbonate. Class 1 antiarrhythmic agents should not be used.
  • Hypotension may require vasopressors/inotropes.
  • Seizures may resolve untreated, but if needed, benzodiazepines and other anticonvulsants can be used.
  • Lipid therapy (intralipid) may have a role in treating refractory TCA overdose.

Selective serotonin re-uptake inhibitors (SSRIs)
Second-generation antidepressants (e.g. citalopram, fluoxetine (Prozac), paroxetine, sertraline).

Mode of action:
> Increase levels of the neurotransmitter serotonin after it is released into the synaptic cleft, by selectively inhibiting SERT on the presynaptic membrane, and preventing its re-uptake. More serotonin is therefore available for entry via the postsynaptic membrane and neurotransmission.

Side effects:
> GI effects (diarrhoea, nausea and vomiting), CNS effects (headaches, drowsiness, agitation), sexual dysfunction, increased risk of bone fractures.
> Suicidal behaviour, particularly in children and adolescents.
> Withdrawal symptoms/discontinuation syndrome if stopped abruptly (especially paroxetine).
> Serotonin syndrome when used with other serotonergic agents.
> Bleeding (especially GI bleeding).

Implications for anaesthesia:
> Continue peri-operatively.
> Drug interactions precipitating serotonin syndrome: linezolid, tramadol, pethidine, methylene blue dye, MOAIs, mirtazapine, TCAs, SNRIs, lithium.
> Inhibition of cytochrome P450 enzymes increases levels of drugs metabolised in the liver (warfarin, theophylline, phenytoin, benzodiazepines).

> Increased risk of GI and post-operative bleeding (inhibits cytochrome P450 potentiating effects of warfarin and impairs platelet function increasing bleeding in patients on antiplatelet agents, NSAIDs and those with liver disease).

Serotonin–norepinephrine re-uptake inhibitors (SNRIs)
Second-generation antidepressants. Examples include venlafaxine and duloxetine.

Mode of action:
> Selectively block SERT and NET at presynaptic membrane, allowing increased levels of serotonin and norepinephrine to enter postsynaptic membrane and promote neurotransmission.

Side effects:
> Dose-dependent hypertension.
> Common side effects on GI and CNS as per SSRIs.

Implications for anaesthesia:
> Continue peri-operatively.
> May potentiate effects of warfarin.
> Drug interactions may cause serotonin syndrome as above, and should be avoided.

Tetracyclic antidepressants (TeCAs)
Examples include mianserin and mirtazapine.

Mode of action:
> Promote noradrenergic and serotonergic neurotransmission via α_2 antagonism.

Side effects:
> Sedation and weight gain due to blockade of various postsynaptic 5-HT_2 receptors.
> Drug interactions – cytochrome P450 enzyme inhibitors and inducers can increase levels or reduce efficacy respectively.

Implications for anaesthesia:
> Continue peri-operatively.

Lithium
Mood stabiliser used in the management of bipolar disorder.

Mode of action:
> Its specific mood-stabilising mechanism remains unclear.
> It can promote the release of serotonin.

Side effects:
> GI (nausea, vomiting, diarrhoea) and CNS (headache, sedation, tremors, hyper-reflexia).
> Hypothyroidism
> Narrow therapeutic index, risk of lithium toxicity (plasma levels >1.5 mmol/L). Signs include – CNS: sedation, confusion, tremors, muscle weakness and slurred speech; CVS: sinus bradycardia, sinus node dysfunction, AV block, T wave changes, hypotension and ventricular irritability.

Implications for anaesthesia:

> Risk of lithium toxicity is high, especially when renal excretion is impaired. Lithium should be discontinued 72 hours prior to surgery (except minor surgery under local anaesthesia) and restarted once electrolytes and haemodynamics are stable.
> Inhibits release of brainstem neurotransmitters reducing requirement for anaesthetic agents.
> Prolongs neuromuscular blockade so neuromuscular monitoring advised.
> Drug interactions increasing lithium levels: NSAIDs, loop and thiazide diuretics, ACE inhibitors.
> ECG monitoring due to risk of various cardiovascular abnormalities.

What is serotonin syndrome?

This is a potentially life-threatening adverse drug reaction, resulting from increased levels of serotonin in the brain stem and spinal cord. A large number of drugs (and their combinations) have been implicated in the serotonin syndrome, including SSRIs, MAOIs, TCAs, pethidine, tramadol and dextromethorphan, linezolid, lithium. It can also occur in SSRI overdose.

Clinical features of this syndrome include:

> Changes in behaviour (agitation and confusion),
> Increased motor activity (muscle rigidity, hyper-reflexia and clonus),
> Autonomic instability (hyperthermia, tachycardia, labile blood pressure and diarrhoea).
> Seizures, rhabdomyolysis, renal failure, arrhythmias, coma and death may occur.
> It may mimic the neuroleptic malignant syndrome.

Treatment is mainly supportive, usually requiring intensive care.

36. DRUGS USED TO TREAT ASTHMA

Asthma is a common disease characterised by reversible airway obstruction secondary to bronchoconstriction. It is a potentially life-threatening condition causing approximately three deaths per day in the UK.

Anaesthetists will regularly anaesthetise patients with asthma and also be involved in the management of the patient with severe or life-threatening asthma. Thus, a thorough understanding of the pathophysiology of asthma and its treatment is expected.

Describe the pathophysiology of severe and life-threatening asthma.

> Bronchospasm from a combination of bronchial smooth muscle constriction, inflammation and mucus production.
> Common triggers include allergens (e.g. house dust mite), tobacco smoke, cold air, exercise, viral infection and, in some patients, drugs such as non-steroidal anti-inflammatory drugs or β-blockers.
> Bronchoconstriction is mediated by the parasympathetic nervous system – acetylcholine released from vagal afferent nerve endings leads to a rise in cyclic cellular calcium levels, causing bronchial smooth muscle contraction.
> Bronchoconstriction results in increased airways resistance and reduced expiratory gas flow, leading to dynamic hyperinflation of the lungs and the generation of intrinsic positive airway pressure.
> Type 1 respiratory failure ensues in the early stages of an acute episode primarily due to ventilation–perfusion mismatching; however, type 2 respiratory failure may develop as the patient becomes exhausted from the increased work of breathing. This is a very ominous sign.

Outline the pharmacological management of asthma.

The aim of pharmacological management of asthma is disease control as defined by absence of symptoms, no limitations on activities and normal lung function. A step-wise approach is adopted, with therapy titrated to severity:

> **Step 1:** Mild intermittent asthma – inhaled short-acting B_2 agonist (e.g. salbutamol) as required.
> **Step 2:** Regular preventative therapy – add inhaled steroid 200–800 µg/day.
> **Step 3:** Initial add-on therapy – add inhaled long-acting B_2 agonist (e.g. salmeterol).

> Assess response and if good then continue. If improvement seen but control still inadequate, increase inhaled steroid dose. If no improvement seen, discontinue long acting B_2 agonist and increase inhaled steroid and consider other therapies such as leukotriene receptor antagonist (e.g. montelukast) or slow-release theophylline.

Leukotriene receptor antagonists block the bronchoconstricting effects of leukotrienes on the airways and act synergistically with inhaled steroids. This class of drug is especially of benefit in exercise-induced asthma. Churg–Strauss syndrome (eosinophilia, vasculitic rash, pulmonary infiltrates) is a rare association with the use of leukotriene receptor antagonists.

> **Step 4:** Persistent poor control – consider trial of increasing inhaled steroid, addition of a fourth drug, e.g. leukotriene receptor antagonist, slow release theophylline or β_2 agonist tablet.
> **Step 5:** Continuous or frequent use of oral steroid – refer to specialist care.

Discuss the drug treatment of severe and life-threatening asthma.

Treatment of severe and life-threatening asthma involves correcting the hypoxaemia and reduction of airways resistance through bronchodilation.

1 **Oxygen** – initially commence high-concentration oxygen and then titrate to maintain $S_aO_2 > 92\%$. Hypoxia is the most common cause of death in life-threatening asthma.

2 **α_2 receptor agonists (nebulised)** – oxygen-driven nebulisation of salbutamol 2.5–5.0 mg back-to-back initially. Drug delivered to the bronchioles is only a small percentage of the total administered dose, due to bronchoconstriction.

3 **Muscarinic antagonist (nebulised)** – oxygen-driven nebulisation of ipratropium bromide 500 μg 6 hourly.

4 **Steroids** – depending on the clinical situation administer either 40 mg prednisolone orally or 200 mg hydrocortisone intravenously followed by 50–100 mg hydrocortisone 6 hourly.

5 **Magnesium sulphate** – administer 2 g over 20 min intravenously. Side effects can include hypotension and muscle weakness however, being an excellent smooth muscle dilator it has an important role in the management of asthma.

6 **Intravenous α_2 agonist** – salbutamol may be administered as an infusion at a rate of 5–20 μg/min, but this is not without potential serious systemic effects such as severe tachycardia and lactic acidosis.

7 **Intravenous phosphodiesterase inhibitor** – aminophylline loading dose of 5 mg/kg followed by an infusion at 0.5 mg/kg/min. Omit the loading dose in those patients already taking oral theophylline (narrow therapeutic index). Aminophylline acts by blocking the enzyme phosphodiesterase thereby increasing intracellular levels of cyclic AMP, which reduces intracellular calcium within the bronchial smooth muscle leading to bronchodilation. Plasma aminophylline levels should be monitored during its use.

8 **Adrenaline** – an excellent bronchodilator through its β agonist action. It should be considered in resistant bronchospasm. It may be administered via nebulisation (1:1000 adrenaline) or in extremis via the intravenous route (titrated 100 μg intravenous boluses).

9 **Heliox** – a mixture of helium and oxygen (commonly 30% oxygen/70% helium). The low density of this gas mixture theoretically improves gas flow within the airways by converting turbulent flow to laminar flow, thereby reducing work of breathing. There is no evidence that it improves outcomes and its use in asthma is no longer recommended by the British Thoracic Society.

10 **Ketamine** – an NMDA receptor antagonist with excellent bronchodilating properties. It may be used to induce anaesthesia in patients with life-threatening asthma and may be used for sedation and treatment of bronchoconstriction in ventilated patients.

11 **Inhalational volatile anaesthetics** – sevoflurane is a good bronchodilator and may be used in resistant bronchospasm. Delivery usually requires an anaesthetic machine although it may be administered through in-line devices in certain critical care ventilators. Gas analysis and scavenging are essential requirements when using volatile agents.

Which drugs should be avoided in acute severe/life-threatening asthma?

> β-Blockers.
> NSAIDs.
> Caution with thiopentone, which may cause histamine release.
> Avoid atracurium, which causes histamine release.
> Caution with morphine, which causes histamine release.

Salbutamol

USES
- Asthma
- COPD
- Hyperkalaemia
- Uncomplicated pre-term labour

ABSORPTION/ DISTRIBUTION
- Extensive first-pass metabolism
- Protein binding 8–64%
- V_D 156 L/kg

MOA
- Direct stimulation of β_2 receptors
- Less pronounced action at β_1 receptors

EFFECTS
CVS
- ↓ BP (β_2)
- At high dose β_1 effects cause ↑ HR and contractility

RS
- Bronchodilation (β_2)
- Reduces hypoxic pulmonary vasoconstriction so can worsen shunt. Always give nebs with O_2

OTHER
- ↓ Uterine tone
- Hypokalaemia – Na^+/K^+ ATPase stimulated transporting K^+ into cells
- ↑ Blood glucose and fatty acids
- Causes skeletal muscle
- Anxiety
- Sweating
- Potentiates non-depolarising muscle relaxants

METABOLISM AND EXCRETION
- Hepatic metabolism
- Metabolites and unchanged drug excreted in urine

SALBUTAMOL
β_2 agonist some small β_1 activity
- Clear colourless solution: 50–500 µg/mL
- Metered dose inhaler: 100 µg, 2 puffs prn
- Powder for inhalation: 200–400 µg, 2 puffs prn
- Liquid 2.5/5 mg/mL for nebulising, prn, titrate to symptoms
- Tablets: 2/4/8 mg, 2–4 mg t.d.s.
- Syrup: 0.4 mg/mL, 2–4 mg t.d.s.

DOSE
- Run infusion at 5–20 µg/min. Titrate to effect

CHEMICAL PROPERTIES
- Nil

Aminophylline

USES
- Asthma
- COPD
- Hyperkalaemia
- Uncomplicated pre-term labour

ABSORPTION/ DISTRIBUTION
- Oral bioavailability up to 96%
- Rectal absorption unpredictable
- Protein binding 50–60%
- V_D 0.4–0.5 L/kg

MOA
- Direct stimulation of β_2 receptors
- Less pronounced action at β_1 receptors

EFFECTS
CVS
- ↑ HR
- ↑ CO
- ↓ SVR
- Arrhythmogenic in higher doses

RS
- Bronchodilation
- ↑ Diaphragmatic contractility
- ↑ Central sensitivity to pCO_2
- Synergistic with β_2 stimulants

CNS
- ↓ Seizure threshold
- ↓ Cerebral blood flow
- Syndrome of inappropriate antidiuretic hormone (SIADH)

RENAL
- Weakly diuretic – inhibits tubular Na^+ reabsorption

AMINOPHYLLINE
Methylxanthine derivative
- Tablets: 100/225/350 mg
- Suppositories: 180/360 mg
- Clear colourless solution: 25 mg/mL

DOSE
- Oral: 900 mg in 2–3 divided doses
- Rectal: 360 mg od
- IV Loading: 5 mg/kg over 10 min (do not load if already on oral drug)
- Maintenance: 0.5 mg/kg/hr

METABOLISM AND EXCRETION
- Hepatic metabolism
- Affected by drugs which induce/inhibit P450 enzyme system
- Subject to zero order kinetics at high doses

TOXICITY
- Subject to zero order kinetics at > 35 µg/kg
- Causes tachyarrhythmias, tremor, seizures, nausea and vomiting, rhabdomyolisis
- Must monitor plasma levels

37. MISCELLANEOUS DRUGS

BENZODIAZEPINES

Diazepam

USES
- Tonic-clonic seizures and status epilepticus
- Anxiolysis
- Alcohol withdrawal
- Muscle spasm
- Sedation
- Premed

MOA
- Agonist at the benzodiazepine receptor which is coupled to GABA receptor
- Stimulation causes ↑ frequency of opening of GABA's Cl^- ion channel
- This causes hyperpolarisation and stabilisation of membrane by increasing flux of Cl^- ions into cell

ABSORPTION/ DISTRIBUTION
- Oral bioavailability up to 100% as very lipid soluble
- Protein binding 99%
- V_D 0.8–1.4 L/kg
- Active metabolites have $t_{1/2}$ >100 hours!

EFFECTS
CVS
- Slight, transient ↓ BP
- ↑ Coronary artery vasodilation
- ↓ Myocardial oxygen demand
RS
- ↓ RR
- Apnoea in high doses
CNS
- Anticonvulsant
- Hypnosis
- Sedation
- Anxiolysis
- Amnesia (anterograde)
- ↓ MAC
- Drowsiness
- Ataxia
- Tolerance and dependence

DIAZEPAM
Benzodiazepine
- Tablets: 2/5/10 mg
- IV white solution: 2/4 mg/mL

DOSE
- IV for sedation: 5–20 mg, titrate to effect
- Alcohol withdrawal: 20–30 mg q.d.s., reducing dose regime
- Status epilepticus: 10 mg IV or PR repeated prn

METABOLISM AND EXCRETION
- Hepatic metabolism to active compounds
  - Desmethyldiazepam,
  - Oxazepam and
  - Temazepam
- Metabolites excreted in urine

CHEMICAL PROPERTIES
- Nil

BENZODIAZEPINE

Midazolam

USES
- Sedation
- Anxiolysis
- With morphine for induction of anaesthesia in unstable patients

ABSORPTION/ DISTRIBUTION
- Oral bioavailability ~ 40%
- Protein binding 95%
- High hepatic extraction ratio, so if hepatic blood flow is poor/poor liver function, half-life will increase
- $t_{1/2}$ 1–4 hours
- Shorter action than other BDZs because of redistribution

MOA
- Agonist at the benzodiazepine receptor coupled to GABA receptor
- Stimulation causes ↑ frequency of opening of GABA's Cl⁻ ion channel
- Causes hyperpolarisation of membrane by increasing flux of Cl⁻ ions into cell

EFFECTS
CVS
- ↓ SVR by one-third
- ↑ HR
- Obtunds response to laryngoscopy when combined with opioid

RS
- ↑ RR
- ↓ V_T
- No change in MV
- Apnoea in some
- Blunts response to pCO_2

CNS
- Hypnosis
- Sedation
- Anxiolysis
- Amnesia (anterograde)
- ↓ Cerebral metabolic oxygen requirements
- ↓ Cerebral blood flow
- ↓ MAC by 15%

GI
- ↓ Hepatic blood flow

GU
- ↓ Renal blood flow

METABOLISM AND EXCRETION
- Hepatic metabolism
- Hydroxylation to 1α hydroxymidazolam (active). This is conjugated and excreted in urine
- <5% converted to oxazepam
- Alfentanil metabolised by same enzymes (P4503A3/4) therefore they may potentiate each other's effects

MIDAZOLAM
Imidazolbenzodiazepine
- Clear colourless solution: 1/2/5 mg/mL
- Oral/nasal/PR/IM/IV/ intrathecally/epidural

DOSE
- Oral: 0.5 mg/kg (max 20 mg)
- IV: 0.02–0.1 mg/kg for sedation, titrate to effect
- Spinal: 0.3–2 mg
- Epidural: 0.1–0.2 mg/kg

CHEMICAL PROPERTIES
- Contains tautomeric diazepine ring structure
- The ring can be open or closed depending on ambient pH
  - > 4 ring closed = non-ionised and lipid soluble
  - < 4 ring open = ionised and less lipid soluble
- pH in ampoule = 3
- pK_a = 8.5 so at pH 7.4, 89% un-ionised
- Drug is water soluble, so no pain on injection
- Effects can be reversed with flumazenil

BENZODIAZEPINE

Temazepam

USES
- Sedation – especially for insomnia
- Anxiolysis
- Pre–med

MOA
- Agonist at benzodiazepine receptor coupled to GABA receptor
- Stimulation causes ↑ frequency of opening of GABA's Cl^- ion channel
- Causes hyperpolarisation of membrane by increasing flux of Cl^- ions into cell

EFFECTS
CVS
- Minimal
RS
- Blunts response to pCO_2 at high doses
CNS
- Hypnosis
- Sedation
- Anxiolysis

ABSORPTION/ DISTRIBUTION
- Oral bioavailability ∼100%
- Protein binding 76%
- V_D 0.8 L/kg
- $t_{1/2}$ 5–11 hours

TEMAZEPAM
Benzodiazepine
- Tablets: 10 mg
- Oral solution: 2 mg/mL

DOSE
- 10–40 mg at night

METABOLISM AND EXCRETION
- Hepatic metabolism
- No significant active metabolites
- Excreted in urine (main route) and faeces

CHEMICAL PROPERTIES
- Nil

Flumazenil

USES
- To reverse effects of benzodiazepines, e.g. if taken in overdose or administered in excess

ABSORPTION/ DISTRIBUTION
- Significant first-pass metabolism
- Protein binding 50%
- V_D 0.9 L/kg
- $t_{1/2}$ 53 min

MOA
- Competitive antagonist at benzodiazepine receptors

EFFECTS
CNS
- Can precipitate seizures
- Can reduce post–operative shivering

FLUMAZENIL
Imidazobenzodiazepine
- Clear, colourless solution: 100 µg/mL

DOSE
- 100 µg boluses. Titrate to effect, max = 1 mg
- Works in 1 min, lasts 15 min–2 hours
- Can give as infusion at 100–400 µg/hr as half-life of benzodiazepine taken in overdose may be longer

METABOLISM AND EXCRETION
- Hepatic metabolism
- No significant active metabolites
- Excreted in urine

CHEMICAL PROPERTIES
- Nil

VASOPRESSORS AND INOTROPES

Phenylephrine

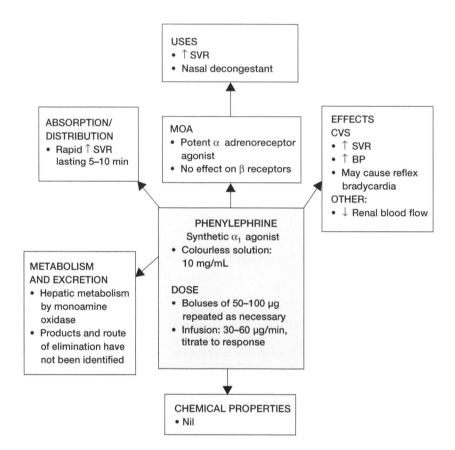

USES
- ↑ SVR
- Nasal decongestant

ABSORPTION/
DISTRIBUTION
- Rapid ↑ SVR
  lasting 5–10 min

MOA
- Potent α adrenoreceptor
  agonist
- No effect on β receptors

EFFECTS
CVS
- ↑ SVR
- ↑ BP
- May cause reflex
  bradycardia
OTHER:
- ↓ Renal blood flow

PHENYLEPHRINE
Synthetic α_1 agonist
- Colourless solution:
  10 mg/mL

DOSE
- Boluses of 50–100 μg
  repeated as necessary
- Infusion: 30–60 μg/min,
  titrate to response

METABOLISM
AND EXCRETION
- Hepatic metabolism
  by monoamine
  oxidase
- Products and route
  of elimination have
  not been identified

CHEMICAL PROPERTIES
- Nil

VASOPRESSORS AND INOTROPES

Metaraminol

USES
- Hypotension
- In treatment of priapism (off licence use)

ABSORPTION/ DISTRIBUTION
- IV administration
- Dose effective within 1–2 min
- Lasts 20–60 min

MOA
- Potent sypathomimetic amine
- Direct stimulation of α_1 and some β receptors – α effects predominate

METABOLISM AND EXCRETION
- Hepatic metabolism

METARAMINOL
Mainly α_1 agonist
some β activity
- Clear colourless solution: 10 mg/mL

DOSE
- Cautious boluses of 0.5 mg, titrate to effect
- Can be run as infusion, tritrate to effect

CHEMICAL PROPERTIES
- Nil

EFFECTS
CVS
- ↑ SVR (this may ↓ CO)
- ↑ BP
- ↑ Coronary artery blood flow
- ↑ Pulmonary artery pressure and vascular resistance
RS
- ↑ RR
- ↑ V_T
OTHER
- ↓ Uterine blood flow
- Uterine contraction therefore, avoid in pregnancy
- ↓ CNS blood flow
- Inhibits insulin release and glycogenolysis causes hyperglycaemia
- ↑ Lipolysis
- ↑ Basal metabolic rate and temperature
SIDE-EFFECTS
- Severe hypertension
- Nausea and vomiting
- Tissue necrosis with extravasation

VASOPRESSORS AND INOTROPES

Noradrenaline

USES
- By infusion to maintain BP and SVR (especially in sepsis)

MOA
- Direct and indirect α_1 agonist
- Some small action at β receptors

ABSORPTION/ DISTRIBUTION
- V_D 0.09–0.4 L/kg

EFFECTS
CVS
- ↑ BP and SVR (CO may ↓)
- Peripheral vasoconstriction
- ↑ Myocardial O_2 consumption
- Coronary artery vasodilation
- ↑ Pulmonary vascular resistance

In excess:
- Hypertenison
- Bradycardia
- Headache
- Peripheral ischaemia

GI
- ↓ Renal blood flow
- ↓ Splanchnic blood flow

CAUTION!
- Contraindicated in patients on MAOIs

METABOLISM AND EXCRETION
- Exogenous noradrenaline: metabolised by:
  - Mitochondrial monoamine oxidase (in liver, brain and kidney)
  - Cytoplasmic COMT
- Excreted in urine, main product is VMA (3-methoxy, 4-hydroxymandelic acid)
- Endogenous noradrenaline metabolised by:
  - Uptake 1: active uptake back in to nerve terminals where reused, or metabolised by MAO
  - Uptake 2: diffusion away from the nerve and metabolised by COMT to VMA, or normetadrenaline

NORADRENALINE
Naturally occurring catecholamine
$\alpha > \beta$ agonist
- Clear colourless solution: 2 mg/mL for dilution

DOSE
- Infusion via central vein: from 0.01 µg/kg/min, titrate to effect

CHEMICAL PROPERTIES
- Give through central vein as highly irritating

VASOPRESSORS AND INOTROPES

Ephedrine

USES
- Hypotension
- Nasal decongestant
- Nocturnal enuresis

MOA
- Indirect sypathomimetic, i.e. causes release of noradrenaline from nerve terminals
- Direct stimulation of α and β receptors
- Inhibits monoamine oxidase

ABSORPTION/ DISTRIBUTION
- Well absorbed PO/IM/SC
- $t_{1/2}$ 4 hours

EFFECTS
CVS
- ↑ HR
- ↑ CO
- ↑ BP
- ↑ Coronary artery blood flow
- ↑ Myocardial O_2 consumption
RS
- Bronchodilation
- ↑RR
GI
- ↓ Renal blood flow
- ↓ GFR
OTHER
- Caution with MAOIs can precipitate hypertensive crisis NB Tachyphylaxis occurs as noradrenaline stores are depleted. Usually seen after ∼ 30 mg given

EPHEDRINE
α and β agonist
- Tablets: 15/30/60 mg
- Clear colourless solution: 30 mg/mL
- Elixir: 3 mg/mL
- Nasal drops: 0.5/1%

DOSE
- Oral: 30 mg t.d.s.
- IV: given as boluses of 3 mg, titrate to effect

METABOLISM AND EXCRETION
- Minimal hepatic metabolism
- 65% excreted unchanged in urine

CHEMICAL PROPERTIES
- Nil

VASOPRESSORS AND INOTROPES

Adrenaline

USES
- In cardiac arrest ALS algorhythm
- Anaphylaxis
- Inotrope
- Nebulised in upper airway obstruction
- Infiltration with local anaesthetic to decrease bleeding

EFFECTS
CVS
Low Dose – β effects predominate
- ↑ CO
- ↑ Cardiac oxygen consumption
- Coronary artery vasodilation
- ↓ Diastolic BP
- ↓ Peripheral vascular resistance
High Dose – α effects predominate
- ↑ SVR
RS
- Potent bronchodilator
- Slight ↑ minute volume
- ↑ Pulmonary vascular resistance
CNS
- ↑ MAC
- ↑ Peripheral pain threshold
GI
- ↓ Splanchnic blood flow
GU
- ↓ Renal blood flow
- ↑ Bladder sphincter tone
METABOLIC
- ↑ BMR
- ↑ Glycogenolysis and plasma glucose
- ↑ Initial insulin secretion (β effect) followed by reduction (α effect)
- ↑ Glucagon secretion
- ↑ Lactate
- ↑ Lipase causing fatty acid oxidation and ketogenesis
- ↑ Renin and aldosterone secretion

ABSORPTION/ DISTRIBUTION
- Inactivated if given orally
- $t_{1/2}$ 2 min

MOA
- α and β adrenoreceptor agonist

ADRENALINE
Naturally occurring catecholamine
α and β agonist
- Clear colourless solution: 0.1–1 mg/mL for IV/IM injection/ nebulisation
- In combination with local anaesthetic at 1:80 000 or 1:200 000

DOSE
- Infusion: 0.01–0.1 µg/kg/min
- 1 mg IV in ALS protocol

METABOLISM AND EXCRETION
- By mitochondrial monoamine oxidase (MAO) and catechol-O-methyl transferase (COMT) in liver, kidney and blood
- Inactive products 3-methoxy-4-hydroymandelic acid (vanillylmandelic acid or VMA) and metadrenaline
- Excreted in urine

CHEMICAL PROPERTIES
- Nil

VASOPRESSORS AND INOTROPES

Dobutamine

USES
- Inotrope in low cardiac output states, e.g. sepsis, post MI
- Cardiac stress testing

ABSORPTION/ DISTRIBUTION
- Dose effective within 1–2 min
- V_D 0.2 L/kg

MOA
- Direct stimulation β receptors

DOBUTAMINE
Synthetic β agonist
$\beta_1 > \beta_2$
- Clear colourless solution: 12.5/50 mg/mL

DOSE
- 0.5–40 µg/kg/min. Titrate to effect

METABOLISM AND EXCRETION
- Hepatic metabolism via COMT
- Inactive metabolites excreted in urine

EFFECTS
CVS
β_1 EFFECTS
- ↑ HR (SA and AV conduction enhanced)
- ↑ Contractility
- ↑ CO
- ↑ Myocardial O_2 demand
- SVR can fall because of dilating effects of β_2 stimulation. May be desirable effect to offload failing heart, or co-administration of noradrenaline may be necessary to maintain SVR
- May precipitate arrhythmias
GI
- Urine output may ↑ with ↑ CO
- No effect on splanchnic vessels
OTHER
- Hypoglycaemia

CHEMICAL PROPERTIES
- Nil

VASOPRESSORS AND INOTROPES

Dopamine

USES
- Inotrope
- Diuretic

MOA
- Low ('renal') dose (1–5 µg/kg/min stimulates D_1 and D_2 receptors
- Higher doses stimulate α and β also
  - 5–10 µg/kg/min mainly β effects
  - 10–20 µg/kg/min mainly α effects

ABSORPTION/ DISTRIBUTION
- Works in 5 min
- Effects last 10 min

DOPAMINE
Naturally occurring catecholamine and neurotransmitter
D_1 and D_2
- Clear colourless solution: 200/800 mg in 5 mL

DOSE
- 1–20 µg/kg/min

METABOLISM AND EXCRETION
- Metabolism via COMT in liver, kidney, plasma. 75% converted to inactive metabolites which are excreted in urine
- 25% converted to noradrenaline in nerves

EFFECTS
CVS
< 5 µg/min – D_1 receptors
- $\downarrow$ Renal vessel resistance $\uparrow$ renal blood flow
< 10 µg/min – $\beta 1$ receptors
- $\uparrow$ HR
- $\uparrow$ Contractility
- $\uparrow$ CO
- $\uparrow$ Coronary artery blood flow
> 10 µg/min – α effects
- $\uparrow$ SVR
RS
- $\downarrow$ Response to hypoxia
AS
- Splanchnic dilation
CNS
- Modulates extrapyramidal movement
- Nausea and vomiting from stimulation of chemoreceptor trigger zone
EXTRA
- Diuretic effect thought to be due to $\uparrow$ CO and by inhibition of Na^+/K^+ ATPase

CHEMICAL PROPERTIES
- Nil

VASOPRESSORS AND INOTROPES

Dopexamine

USES
- Inotrope
- To ↑ splanchnic and renal perfusion

MOA
- Direct stimulation of dopaminergic receptors
- Direct stimulation of β_2 receptors
- Inhibits uptake-1 of noradrenaline

ABSORPTION/ DISTRIBUTION
- 40% bound to red blood cells
- V_D 0.3–0.45 L/kg

EFFECTS
CVS
- ↑ HR
- ↑ Contractility
- ↑ CO (helped by ↓ afterload)
- Improved coronary artery perfusion with no increase in myocardial O_2 demand
- Rarely precipitates arrhythmias
GI
- ↑ Renal blood flow causes diuresis
- ↑ Splanchnic blood flow
RS
- Bronchodilation (β_2)
OTHER
- Hyperglycaemia (β_2)
- Hypokalaemia (β_2)
- Nausea and vomiting from D_2 effect at CTZ
NB Avoid in fixed cardiac output states or phaeochromocytoma

DOPEXAMINE
Synthetic β_2, D_1 and D_2 agonist
- Clear colourless solution: 10 mg/mL

DOSE
- 0.5–6 μg/kg/min. Titrate to effect

METABOLISM AND EXCRETION
- Hepatic metabolism
- Metabolites excreted in urine and faeces

CHEMICAL PROPERTIES
- Nil

β AGONIST

Isoprenaline

USES
- Holding measure in complete heart block while awaiting pacing (temporary or permanent)
- Inotrope

ABSORPTION/ DISTRIBUTION
- Well absorbed orally
- Extensive first-pass metabolism
- Low bioavailability

MOA
- Potent β_1 and β_2 adrenoreceptor agonist
- No α effects

EFFECTS
CVS
β_1
- ↑ HR
- ↑ Contractility
- ↑ CO
β_2
- Can ↓ SVR negating any rise in BP caused by ↑ CO
- Can ↓ coronary artery perfusion as diastolic filling time reduced
RS
- Potent bronchodilator (but not used in asthma as there is an associated rise in mortality)
CNS
- Stimulant
GI
- ↑ Mesenteric and renal blood flow
Metabolic
- ↑ Blood glusoe and free fatty acids

METABOLISM AND EXCRETION
- Hepatic metabolism by catechol-O-methlytransferase
- Metabolites and large amount of unchanged drug excreted in urine

ISOPRENALINE
Synthetic β_1 and β_2 agonist
- Tablets: 30 mg
- Colourless solution: 0.02 or 1 mg/mL
- Metered dose aerosol: 80/400 μg

DOSE
- Oral: 30 mg t.d.s.
- IV: 0.5–8 μg/min, titrate to effect. Takes ~ 20 min to take effect

CHEMICAL PROPERTIES
- Nil

VASOPRESSORS AND INOTROPES

Milrinone

USES
• Inotrope
• Low cardiac output states especially following cardiac surgery

MOA
• Inhibits PDE III and therefore reduces degradation of cAMP in cardiac and smooth muscle
• ↑ cAMP increases intracellular release of Ca^{2+}, therefore increasing biventricular contractility
• Alters Ca^{2+} flux into smooth muscles causing relaxation of vessels, including pulmonary vasodilatation

ABSORPTION/ DISTRIBUTION
• Protein binding 70%
• V_D 0.45 L/kg
• $t_{1/2}$ 2.5 hours

EFFECTS
CVS
• ↑ Stroke volume
• ↑ Contractility
• ↑ Cardiac index
• No increase in cardiac oxygen consumption
• ↓ SVR
• ↑ Pulmonary vasodilatation
• Can cause hypotension
• Less tachycardia than with β-agonists (e.g. dobutamine)
• Ventricular ectopics, VT and VF reported (rarely)
• Angina
CNS
• Headache
CAUTION!
Slightly increases AV nodal conduction use with care in patients with AF/flutter. Consider co-administration of digoxin if necessary.

MILRINONE
Selective phosphodiesterase III Inhibitor
• Yellow solution: 1 mg/mL

DOSE
• Loading: 50 µg/kg over 10 min
• Maintenance: 0.375–0.75 µg/kg/min

METABOLISM AND EXCRETION
• Hepatic metabolism
• Excreted in urine, 85% unchanged

CHEMICAL PROPERTIES
• Nil

VASOPRESSORS AND INOTROPES

Levosimendan

USES
- Acute decompensated severe congestive cardiac failure

MOA
- Binds to troponin C and stabilises troponin C and actin-myosin cross-bridges
- Therefore, increases contractility and vasodilatation without increasing Ca^{2+} concentration by sensitising cardiac muscle filaments to Ca^{2+}
- Does not increase oxygen or ATP consumption

ABSORPTION/ DISTRIBUTION
- Oral bioavailability 85%
- Protein binding 98%
- $t_{1/2}$ 1 hour

EFFECTS
CVS
- ↑ Stroke volume
- ↑ Contractility
- ↑ Cardiac index
- No increase in cardiac oxygen consumption
- ↓ SVR, PVR and PCWP
- Arrhythmias: AF, atrial and ventricular tachycardias
CNS
- Headache
CAUTION!
Use CI'd in:
- Severe hepatic/renal failure
- Ventricular outflow obstruction
- Severe hypotension/ tachycardia
- History of torsades de pointes

LEVOSIMENDAN
Calcium sensitiser
- Clear colourless solution: 2.5 mg/mL

DOSE
- Loading: 6–12 µg/kg over 10 min
- Maintenance: 0.05–0.2 µg/ kg/min. Single infusion given for 24 hours and then discontinued. Continuing drug does not improve outcomes

METABOLISM AND EXCRETION
- Hepatic metabolism
- Excreted in urine, 85% unchanged

CHEMICAL PROPERTIES
- Nil

UTEROTONICS

Oxytocin

USES
• To cause uterine contraction:
  • Induction of labour
  • Following caesarean section
  • Following abortion

MOA
• Stimulates uterine contraction by binding to specific sites on muscle cells
• Agonist at oxytocin receptor G protein coupled receptor

EFFECTS
GU
• Uterine contraction. Fetal heart rate must be monitored once infusion starts
• Overdose can cause hyperstimulation
• Mild antidiurectic effect, only apparent with prolonged use
CVS
• ↑ SVR
• ↑ BP
• Severe hypertension in patients with cardiac disease
• Tachycardia (marked) follows bolus – give slowly
GI
• Nausea and vomiting
Other
• Rash
• Anaphylaxis
• Amniotic fluid embolism reported following overdose

ABSORPTION/ DISTRIBUTION
• Given IV
• Acts within 2–3 min

OXYTOCIN
Trade name: Syntocinon
Synthetically produced posterior pituitary hormone
• Clear colourless solution: 5 IU/mL

DOSE
• Induction of labour by IV infusion 0.001–0.002 u/min. Do not exceed 5 u per day
• 5 u by *slow* bolus given immediately following delivery of newborn at caesarean section

METABOLISM AND EXCRETION
• Hepatic and renal metabolism

CHEMICAL PROPERTIES
• Octapeptide

UTEROTONICS

Carbetocin

USES
- To cause sustained uterine contraction following caesarean section.
- Can only give 1 dose

MOA
- Agonist at G protein coupled oxytocin receptor and so stimulates uterine contraction.
- Effects seen within 2 mins, last 1 hour.

ABSORPTION/ DISTRIBUTION
- $t_{\frac{1}{2}}$ 85 – 100 mins

EFFECTS
CVS
- Tachycardia Chest pain

RS
- Respiratory distress

CNS
- Dizziness
- Metallic taste

GI
- N&V
- Abdo pain

OTHER
- Itching
- Raised temp
- Sweating
- Chills
- Trembling
- Back pain

CAUTION IN THOSE WITH:
- Hypertension
- IHD

CARBETOCIN
Long acting synthetic analogue of oxytocin

Clear colourless solution 100 µg/mL

CARBETOCIN
- 100 µg IV over 1 min given immediately following parturition.
- Once only dosing
- Uterine contraction sustained for approx. 1 hour (compared to syntocinon = approx. 15 mins)

METABOLISM & EXCRETION
- Mechanism of elimination not known? enzymatic degradation
- Minimally renally excreted (0.7%)

CHEMICAL PROPERTIES
- None

UTEROTONICS

Ergometrine

USES
- To cause uterine contraction and reduce bleeding:
  - Following caesarean section
  - Following abortion
  - Second line treatment of uterine atony after oxytocin / carbetocin

MOA
- Stimulates uterine and vascular smooth muscle contraction? by binding to 5HT receptors
- Stimulates D_2 receptors at chemoreceptor trigger zone (CTZ) causing emesis

EFFECTS
GU
- Uterine contraction follows 1 min after IV and 5 min after IM dosing
CVS
- ↑ SVR and BP
- Severe hypertension. Can be harmful in patients with cardiac disease – lasts several hours
- CI in pre-eclampsia
- Bradycardia and arrhythmias (marked)
- MI reported
- Pulmonary oedema
CNS
- Headache
- Dizziness
- Tinnitus
- CVA reported
GI
- Severe nausea and vomiting

ABSORPTION/ DISTRIBUTION
- Acts within
  - 1 min IV
  - 5 min IM
  - 10 min PO
- Lasts 3–6 hours

ERGOMETRINE
Ergot alkaloid derivative
- Solution: 0.5 mg/mL
- Tablets: 0.5 mg
- Combined with syntocinon (syntometrine): 0.5 mg ergometrine + 5 IU syntocinon/mL for IM injection

DOSE
- 0.5 mg IM or 0.125 mg by slow IV injection. Repeat if necessary

METABOLISM AND EXCRETION
- Hepatic metabolism
- Excreted in bile

CHEMICAL PROPERTIES
- Nil

UTEROTONICS

Carboprost

USES
- To cause uterine contraction and stop post-partum haemorrhage in patients unresponsive to oxytocin and ergometrine

MOA
- Stimulates uterine contraction
- Mechanism not elucidated

EFFECTS
GU
- Uterine contraction
RS
- Bronchospasm – relatively contraindicated in asthmatics
CVS
- Cardiovascular collapse reported
- Pulmonary oedema (rare)
- Sweating
- Flushing
CNS
- Headache
- Dizziness
GI
- Nausea and vomiting

ABSORPTION/ DISTRIBUTION
- No information

CARBOPROST
Prostaglandin $F_{2\alpha}$ analogue
Trade name: Hemabate
- Solution: 250 µg/mL

DOSE
- 250 µg IM or directly into uterine muscle. Repeat every 15 min as necessary
- Max dose 2 g

METABOLISM AND EXCRETION
- No information

CHEMICAL PROPERTIES
- Nil

Part 02

SPECIAL PATIENT GROUPS

38. THE JEHOVAH'S WITNESS

Jehovah's Witnesses (JW) date back to the 1870s and consider themselves a part of the Christian religion. Their text is the 'The New World Translation' of the Bible; they believe that Jesus, the only son of Jehovah, died for our sins, but they do not accept the concept of the Holy Trinity. They maintain political neutrality, believing that only God, not government, should be in the ultimate position of authority, and consequently remain as conscientious objectors during conflict. There are, of course, many facets to the religion beyond the scope of this book, but the one that causes us considerable concern as doctors is the refusal of some JWs to accept the transfusion of blood products. This refusal is results from the words in Genesis 9:3–4, Leviticus 17:11–12, and Acts 15:28–29.

What are Jehovah's Witnesses' beliefs surrounding transfusion of blood products?

A committed JW is forbidden by the scriptures-from receiving blood products. Transgressing this rule compromises their relationship with God and may leave a JW feeling that life is meaningless. Giving blood products to a JW against their will has been likened, by them, to the assault of rape, in terms of its psychological impact. Each competent adult has the right to refuse to give consent to any treatment and does not have to explain their reasons for this refusal. If a doctor wilfully transfuses a JW against their wishes, then he/she is liable to criminal and civil prosecution for assault, and also could be subject to GMC disciplinary proceedings.

Which products are unacceptable?

Unfortunately, there are no hard and fast rules, as each individual will decide which treatments are acceptable to them.

Generally, the following are not acceptable:
> Whole blood
> Packed cells
> White cells
> Platelets
> Fresh frozen plasma
> Autotransfusion of blood that has been taken and stored

The individual will decide about the acceptability of the following:
> Blood salvage
> Dialysis
> Haemodilution
> Cardio-pulmonary bypass (non-blood-primed circuit)
> Blood fractions, e.g. albumin, immunoglobulins, clotting factors
> Transplanted organs
> Epidural blood patches

It is important to discuss beliefs with the individual before planning the anaesthetic, blood loss prevention and rescue strategies.

Patients can discuss the various blood products and strategies with a committee of elders called the 'Hospital Liaison Committee for Jehovah Witnesses'. Each hospital switchboard will have this number.

It is important to document clearly all discussions with the patient. There is a special consent form for JWs, upon which their specific individual wishes must be recorded.

How would you assess a Jehovah's Witness pre-operatively for elective surgery?

> A JW included on a list should be flagged up as soon as possible so that their wishes can be discussed and the best anaesthetic/surgical technique planned.
> A consultant who is happy to anaesthetise JWs should be allocated to the case.
> Clearly, the risk to the individual will be related to the nature of the surgery. It is sensible to discuss the risks with the patient alone, so that they are under no duress from other members of the church when it comes to making decisions about their treatment.
> The decisions made following this consultation must be entered in the notes, dated, timed and signed by both the doctor and the patient. The discussion must be frank and honest, and the consequences of refusing blood or blood products impressed upon the patient.
> Any anaemia should be investigated and treated in a timely manner, where possible. Oral iron may be given (this will not raise Hb acutely), or for some, recombinant erythropoietin is acceptable (though it is not licensed for this use). Discuss cases that are not straightforward with a haematologist.

How would you assess a Jehovah's Witness pre-operatively for emergency surgery?

> The principles of patient care are unchanged here, but there may be uncertainty as to the patient's wishes if they have lost 'capacity' by the time of presentation.
> Many JWs have an advanced directive detailing their wishes. If they are not carrying this, it is often lodged with their GP and efforts should be made to find it.
> If no advanced directive exists, or can be found, for a patient lacking capacity, we must act in the perceived best interests of the patient. This can mean giving blood/blood products if we believe the therapy to be truly life saving. The decision-making process must be documented meticulously, and a consultant must be involved in the decision.

Describe how you would conduct your anaesthetic for a Jehovah's Witness.

The surgical and anaesthetic techniques must be aimed at minimising blood loss. The following options should be considered where appropriate:

> Arterial tourniquets
> Careful positioning
> Hypotensive anaesthesia
> Vasoconstrictors
> Haemodilution
> Meticulous haemostasis
> Optimising clotting – avoid acidosis and maintain normothermia
> Cell salvage, if this is acceptable to the individual and not contraindicated by their condition
> Drugs that promote clotting, e.g. Factor VIIa, tranexamic acid and aprotinin.

It may be sensible to stagger operations to allow for haematological recovery in between each one.

Several operations lend themselves to regional techniques, e.g. caesarean delivery. This can help to reduce blood loss and also, should bleeding become life threatening, the awake patient may have the opportunity to change their mind about receiving blood/blood products.

Are there any special considerations for the post-operative period?

> Monitor ongoing blood loss – surgical re-exploration must not be delayed if bleeding is suspected.
> Patients who have suffered excessive blood loss may need to be electively ventilated in an attempt to optimise their oxygen delivery.
> There are reports of using hyperbaric oxygen therapy in the face of very low haemoglobins, but this is not widely available.

Issues surrounding capacity and consent.

We include this section because these issues are of interest and not well covered in other texts. However, examiners will not expect you to be masters of law. To display an appreciation of the sensitive nature and potential complexity of the issues, and to show appropriate caution and seek senior advice, will be enough to pass.

Children <16 years of age:

By law, this group may give consent to treatment if they are believed to function at a level that allows them to understand the information given them, weigh it in the balance, use it to make a decision and communicate that decision. This is called being 'Gillick-competent', so called because of the legal case brought by Victoria Gillick which turned on the issue of whether a minor may have the capacity to give valid consent. The court believed that they might and consequently, a 'Gillick-competent' child may, in theory, consent to, or refuse, treatment. However, in practical terms, at the time of publication, the courts have never upheld a child's refusal of life-saving treatment, no matter how well reasoned their argument. Applying past case law to the situation in which a child who is a Jehovah's Witness needs a life-saving blood transfusion, it is most likely that the courts will find that the child does not have the capacity to refuse this treatment. Conversely, if a child who is deemed Gillick-competent consents to a blood transfusion, that consent stands even in the face of parental refusal.

If both the parents and the child refuse transfusion, or the child is not Gillick-competent to give consent in the face of parental refusal, the medical team can apply for a 'Special Issue Order' via the High Court. If granted, this will allow the doctors to give treatment. This order must only be sought in non-emergency situations where it is thought that the treatment will prevent serious permanent harm or be life saving. The manager on call for the hospital will have the procedural information for obtaining a 'Special Issue Order'.

In a life-threatening emergency, the child should be treated with whatever means necessary to preserve life, regardless of the parents' wishes.

Children 16–18 years of age:

According to the Mental Capacity Act 2005, patients of 16 years and over can be assumed to have the capacity to make decisions regarding their treatment; however, the parents, rather paradoxically, retain the right to consent for a child until they reach 18 years. This could lead to potential conflict if a patient aged 16–18 years were a JW but their parents were not. Here, a situation could arise in which the child refuses blood/blood products but the parents want them to be transfused. In this case, the law would suggest that the patient is treated as an adult and their choice to refuse respected, provided the patient understands the consequences of their decision. This situation has not yet been tested in the courts and therefore no precedent has been set. Looking to the law for guidance, there is no 'correct answer' to this dilemma. Whatever the decision, there are going to be serious repercussions – either the patient's wishes are ignored and medical therapy commenced or the parents' wishes are ignored and they are left bereaved. If time permitted it would be sensible to seek legal advice on such issues. All decisions must be made at consultant level. All treatment must be given in the best interests of the patient.

The rights of the anaesthetist.

Anaesthetists have the right to refuse to undertake elective anaesthesia on JWs, but are duty-bound to refer such cases to someone with the appropriate expertise, who is willing to be involved.

In emergency situations, anaesthetists are expected to provide care to JWs, and fully abide by their wishes, once these have been verified.

39. OBESITY

Obesity is an increasing problem in the developed world. Consider obesity as a medical problem with associated physiological and patho-physiological consequences.

How is obesity classified?

Obesity of classified in terms of the body mass index (BMI).

$$BMI = weight (kg)/height (m^2)$$

BMI	Definition
<18.5	Underweight
18.5–24.9	Ideal weight
25–29.9	Overweight
30–39.9	Obese
40–49.9	Morbidly obese
50–59.9	Super obese
60–69.9	Super super-obese
>70	Hyper-obese

What are the physiological changes associated with obesity that complicate anaesthesia?

> **Airway**
>   • Higher incidence of difficult face mask ventilation and difficult intubation
> **Respiratory**
>   • Increased O_2 consumption and CO_2 production, which may be associated with chronic hypercarbia.
>   • Decreased chest wall compliance causes increased work of breathing.
>   • Decreased functional residual capacity (FRC), especially when supine, means that closing capacity may encroach on FRC; once BMI exceeds 40, FRC falls to 1 L or less.
>   • Increased incidence of obstructive sleep apnoea (OSA).
>   • Obesity hypoventilation syndrome occurs (i.e. low O_2 saturations not caused by obstruction).
>   • Increased incidence of asthma.
>   • Increased incidence of pulmonary hypertension.
>   • These factors result in a high risk of peri-operative hypoxia.
> **Cardiovascular**
>   • Increased blood volume and cardiac output.
>   • Increased incidence of ischaemic heart disease, arrhythmias, hypertension, hyperlipidaemia, heart failure and cor pulmonale.
> **Metabolic**
>   • Increased incidence of type 2 diabetes mellitus.

> **Gastrointestinal**
> • Increased incidence of hiatus hernia, gastro-oesophageal reflux disease, fatty liver and cirrhosis
> • Decreased rate of stomach emptying
> • Raised intra-abdominal pressure, which can cause compartment syndrome
> **Haematology**
> • Higher incidence of venous thromboembolism

What are the pharmacodynamic and pharmacokinetic changes that occur?

> **Pharmacokinetics**
> • Altered volume of drug distribution (V_D) and elimination
> • The use of 'ideal' or 'actual' body weight during drug dose calculation must be considered
> **Ideal body weight in kg**
> • Height (cm) – 100 for adult males
> • Height (cm) – 105 for adult females
> **Volatiles**
> • Sevoflurane and desflurane – pharmacokinetics not significantly altered.
> • Halothane – increased reductive hepatic metabolism, increasing the risk of halothane hepatitis.
> **Induction agents**
> • Thiopentone – increased V_D and longer elimination half-life. Suggested dose is 7.5 mg/kg based on ideal body weight.
> • Propofol – induction dose should be based on ideal body weight. When used for maintenance (TIVA), calculate dose using actual body weight, as propofol does not accumulate in obese patients.
> **Opioids**
> • Fentanyl – pharmacokinetics not altered, use actual body weight.
> • Morphine – accumulates in body fat, use ideal body weight.
> **Muscle relaxants**
> • Suxamethonium – use actual body weight.
> • Rocuronium – use ideal body weight.

What are the anaesthetic considerations for an obese patient presenting for surgery?

> **Pre-operative assessment**
> • When planning elective surgery, pre-operative assessment should involve a multi-disciplinary team.
> • Ensure sufficient time is allocated for the patient on the operating list. Both the anaesthetic and surgery are likely to be technically more difficult and take longer.
> • Assess and establish co-morbidities to help define 'risk'. This will be dependent on the individual patient and the proposed surgery. The severity of symptoms, e.g. angina, may be masked by a sedentary lifestyle. Request further investigation as appropriate, e.g. lung function tests, ECHO.
> • Anaesthetic history, including thorough airway assessment, grade of previous intubations and patient's ability to lie flat, if necessary.
> • Consider regional techniques where possible.
> • Optimise the patient for surgery if possible, e.g. weight loss programme and optimisation of medical conditions.
> • Liaise with critical care to arrange appropriate post-operative care, e.g. HDU/ICU and non-invasive ventilation.
> • Ensure a senior anaesthetist is available for the case.
> • Inform theatres in advance to ensure bariatric equipment is available (e.g. electric bed, operating table, hover mattress and large blood pressure cuffs).

> **Induction**
  - Pre-medicate with antacid prophylaxis or a proton pump inhibitor.
  - If possible, get the patient to climb onto the operating table and position themselves. If not, use aids such as a hover mattress.
  - Anticipate difficult intravenous access and use ultrasound if necessary.
  - Have a low threshold for invasive blood pressure monitoring, as cuffs can be inaccurate.
  - Position the patient 30° head up.
  - Consider awake fibre-optic intubation.
  - Use a short-handle laryngoscope with a long blade and ensure the difficult airway trolley is available.
  - Ensure strict pre-oxygenation (end-tidal oxygen >90%).

> **Maintenance**
  - Use short-acting anaesthetic agents, e.g. desflurane, sevoflurane, propofol, remifentanil.
  - Ventilate using PEEP.
  - Ensure pressure areas are padded and monitored.
  - Ensure adequate fluid input given larger surface area of patient.
  - Monitor and maintain temperature.

> **Post-operative management**
  - Ensure there are sufficient people present to move the patient safely.
  - Extubate awake and sitting up. Consider extubating onto CPAP.
  - Prescribe supplementary O_2 for at least 24 hours post-operatively.
  - Admit to a suitable level of care, based on your assessment of risk.
  - Thromboprophylaxis.
  - Multimodal analgesia.
  - Early physiotherapy and mobilisation.

Obese patients are some of the most challenging patients to anaesthetise, and your answer should reflect the difficulties they can present.

40. PAEDIATRIC PATIENT

Children are not small adults. Paediatric patients vary considerably and include the following groups:

> *Premature – less than 37 weeks post-conception*
> *Neonate – first 28 days of life or <44 weeks post-conception*
> *Infant – 1 month to 1 year*
> *Child – >1 year to 12 years*
> *Adolescent – 13 to 16 years*

The differences between paediatric and adult anaesthetic practice reduce as the patients become older. The important anatomical and physiological differences have been covered in Study Guide 1, *Chapter 36, 'Child versus adult'.*

What are the major anaesthetic considerations for the paediatric patient?

Pre-operative visit:

> This is an important time to develop trust and rapport with the child and parent. A friendly, calm and reassuring approach will help alleviate parental and child anxiety.
> Take a medical and anaesthetic history. This should cover the following:
> * Preterm/term baby
> * Developmental milestones
> * Medical conditions including congenital anomalies
> * Recent respiratory illness
> * Current medication
> * Recent immunisations
> * Allergies
> * Any previous problems with anaesthetics including family history
> * Loose teeth
> * Fasting times
> Explain the planned approach to induction so both parent and child know what to expect. For a gas induction it is important to inform parents of the 'excitatory' phase of the induction and explain that their child may wriggle and try and push the mask away but that this phase is only transient and the child will have no explicit recollection of the event.
> Gain consent for suppositories.
> Explain post-operative pain management.
> Obtain the weight of the child, as all drug doses and airway devices are based on weight.

Approximate estimates of weight under 1 year are:
> Neonates: 3–3.5 kg
> 3 months: 6 kg
> 6 months: 7–8 kg
> 9 months: 9 kg
> 12 months: 10 kg

For children aged between 1 year and 10 years, weight can be estimated using the formula:

$$\text{Weight (kg)} = (\text{Age} + 4) \times 2$$

This is the standard formula that is universally used. However, newer formulas exist to adjust for the fact that children are now getting heavier.

Children 1–5 years: Weight = (Age × 2) + 8
Children 6–12 years: Weight = (Age × 3) + 7

> Consider pre-medication.
>   • Oral sedative pre-medication (e.g. midazolam) is now infrequently used routinely. It is useful in children who are very anxious or who are likely to be uncooperative. To work effectively, it needs be given 30 minutes in advance and therefore the list needs to be planned accordingly. Buccal midazolam is gaining popularity as its onset time is quicker than the oral formulation (20 minutes).
>   • Analgesic pre-medication is becoming more routinely used now (e.g. paracetamol and ibuprofen).
>   • EMLA or amethocaine (Ametop) cream should be applied to identifiable veins if an intravenous induction is planned.
> Conduct a targeted physical examination if required.
> Investigations are rarely required but on some occasions may be necessary:
>   • Haemoglobin – if large blood loss expected, premature infants, systemic disease or congenital heart disease
>   • Electrolytes – if renal or metabolic disease or dehydration
>   • CXR – if significant active respiratory disease, scoliosis, congenital heart disease

---

Upper respiratory tract infections (URTIs): The decision to postpone or proceed with surgery in a child with an URTI is multifactorial and must take into consideration the child's age, co-morbidities, presenting symptoms, urgency and type of surgery.

> *Children under 1 year – have a low threshold to cancel in this age group as respiratory complications are higher.*
> *If the child appears well, with only clear nasal discharge and no other symptoms, with surgery not involving the airway and the child not requiring intubation – it would be reasonable to proceed with the case.*
> *If the child has purulent nasal discharge, productive cough and/ or fever, or there are clinical signs suggesting lower respiratory tract involvement such as desaturation or wheeze – the case should be postponed for at least 4 weeks.*

Table 40.1 Paediatric fasting times

Fasting time	Food type
6 hours	Solids, cow's milk and formal milk
4 hours	Breast milk
2 hours	Clear fluids

Anaesthetic preparation:

> Prepare your anaesthetic drugs and emergency drugs (e.g. atropine and suxamethonium).
> Drugs are calculated according to the child's weight (*see* Table 40.2 for common paediatric drug doses). You should calculate these in advance and write them down (it is also worth documenting the volume of drug that this represents, e.g. 15 µg fentanyl = 0.3 mL).
> When small volumes of drugs are to be administered, they should be drawn up undiluted in a 1 mL syringe.
> Prepare your airway equipment, breathing circuit (e.g. T-piece) and monitoring in advance and ensure that you have a paediatric Ambu bag with alternative oxygen supply immediately available.
> T-piece breathing circuit is used for patients below 20 kg (Ayre's original form was a Mapleson E system. Jackson Rees modified this later by including an open-ended reservoir bag and using a longer reservoir tube; this is known as the Mapleson F system, or Ayre's T-piece with Jackson Rees modification).
> If small volumes of intravenous fluids are to be administered, a burette should be used.
> Warm the theatre and prepare any warming devices.
> A parent and member of staff usually accompany the child into the anaesthetic room. Some parents may be quite anxious and therefore a positive and empathetic approach can go a long way.

Induction of anaesthesia:

A calm, friendly environment will help reduce anxiety in both the child and parent. The aim is to try and ensure the child does not feel scared. A calm, co-operative child will greatly facilitate the induction process.

> **Inhalational gas induction**
   • This is a good technique for neonates and infants (small and easy to hold), and also for children who fear needles or have difficult venous access.
   • It is a two-person technique, requiring one to perform the gas induction and maintain the airway once the child is anaesthetised and the other to gain intravenous access (which must be done prior to siting an airway due to the risk of laryngospasm).
   • If the child is small, then often a gas induction can be performed with the child sitting on the parent's lap (they will need to be strategically held/cuddled by the parent in order to prevent them from struggling and pushing the mask away). The best approach to anaesthetising neonates and small/premature infants is with the child lying on the trolley once the parents have been escorted from the anaesthetic room/theatre.
   • An oxygen–sevoflurane mix is used (in the past halothane was used). Sevoflurane has a pungent smell but is non-irritant. It has a rapid onset and offset of action. The concentration should ideally be increased gradually in most cases in order to minimise the patients' distress; however, in certain situations (e.g. uncooperative patients) sevoflurane may be dialled up to 8% from the outset. The use of nitrous oxide increases the speed of onset and depth of anaesthesia obtained. MAC values are 3.3 in infants, 2.5 in children and 1.7 in adults. Once anaesthesia is achieved and IV access is secured, air–oxygen mixture should be used as carrier gas.
   • There is often an excitatory phase during the induction and this can worry some parents unless they have been told about it beforehand.
   • There is an 'art' to performing a good gas induction, which can only be gained with experience (pay attention to subtle things, e.g. what side of the parent and child to stand on, how to hold the mask so that it does not look like you are smothering the child, etc.).

> **Intravenous induction:**
>   - This has a rapid and defined end point and may be considered an easier technique by non-paediatric anaesthetists but the caveat to this is gaining intravenous access, which can be challenging, especially in toddlers with chubby little hands and feet. Patients may also desaturate more quickly compared with a gas induction.
>   - The best sites for intravenous access are back of the hand, inner wrist, long saphenous vein and veins on the dorsum of the foot.
>   - Pre-oxygenation can be difficult in small children but should be undertaken if possible, especially if rapid sequence induction is planned.
>   - Propofol, thiopentone or ketamine can all be used.

Airway devices:

> **Intubation**
>   - All infants less than 5 kg or under 44 weeks gestational age should be intubated.
>   - Straight blades (Robertshaw or Miller): use in neonates and infants.
>   - Curved blade: easier to use once the child is 6–10 kg.
>   - For children between the age of 1 year and 10 years, uncuffed endotracheal tube (ETT) internal diameter (ID) size can be estimated using the formula:

$$\text{ETT size} = \text{Age}/4 + 4.5$$
(this is generally a better fit than: Age/4 + 4)

>   - Uncuffed tubes: typically used until 8–10 years of age to minimise the risk of damage to the trachea. A small leak should be present, but if the leak is too large it will compromise ventilation. Modern endotracheal tubes have low-pressure, high-volume cuffs and there are centres that use cuffed tubes in very young children with no complications. Opt for internal diameter 1/2 size smaller when using a cuffed ETT.
>   - Ideally the ETT should be inserted such that its thick black marking is at the level of the vocal cords. Appropriate length can also be calculated as follows:

$$\text{Oral ETT length (in cm)} = \text{Age}/2 + 12$$
$$\text{Nasal ETT length (in cm)} = \text{Age}/2 + 15$$
(or an easier one to remember is oral ETT = ID × 3, for nasal ETT, add 2 cm)

>   - Appropriate ID size and length in neonates is 3–3.5 and 8–10 cm, respectively, and in infants 4–4.5 and 10–12 cm.
>   - Once ETT is inserted, its correct placement should be confirmed with auscultation and $ETCO_2$ monitoring.
>   - Laryngospasm at extubation occurs less frequently if the child is fully awake at the time of extubation.
>   - You may need to be with the child in recovery until fully awake if the recovery staff are inexperienced with children.

> **Laryngeal mask airway**
>   - The size used is based on the weight of the child:
>   - 0–5 kg = size 1
>   - 5–10 kg = size 1.5
>   - 10–20 kg = size 2
>   - 20–30 kg = size 2.5
>   - >30 kg = size 3

Maintenance fluids:

> In 2007 the NPSA released an alert on the risk of hyponatraemia in children receiving intravenous fluids. Since then hypotonic solutions (e.g. 0.18% saline with 4% dextrose) are not to be routinely used in children.
> NICE will release information on intravenous fluids for children in October 2015, which will provide recommendations on the types of fluids that should be used for resuscitation and maintenance purposes.
> Currently, for peri-operative intravenous maintenance fluid, a balanced, isotonic solution should be used.
> Short operations (<1 hour) in healthy children do not usually require fluids if pre-operative fasting has not been excessive.
> Children undergoing intra-abdominal surgery or where there is anticipated blood loss should receive intravenous fluids.
> When calculating peri-operative fluid requirements, fluid lost during the pre-operative fasting period and intra-operative losses should be added to the maintenance fluid requirements.
> Maintenance fluids are calculated as follows:
> • First 10 kg: 4 mL/kg/h (or 100 mL/kg/24 h)
> • Next 10 kg: 2 mL/kg/h (or 50 mL/kg/24 h)
> • Subsequent kg: 1 mL/kg/h (or 20 mL/kg/24 h)
> (so a 9 kg child would have a maintenance fluid requirement of 36 mL/h and a 20 kg child would require 60 mL/h).
> Fluid boluses:
> • Non-resuscitation: 10 mL/kg
> • Resuscitation: 20 mL/kg

Analgesia:

> Add regional analgesia where appropriate (e.g. caudal for urological, inguinal hernia and lower limb procedures, axillary blocks for upper limb surgery).
> Pre-medicate where possible.
> Gain consent for suppositories.
> Do not give codeine to children under the age of 12 years.
> Use a multi-modal approach.

What are the main pharmacokinetic and pharmacodynamic differences?

> Decreased lean body mass.
> Increased total body water (TBW is 85% at birth vs 60% in adult) – so higher initial dose required.
> Decreased total body fat and therefore increased volume of distribution (V_d) for water-soluble drugs. Drugs terminated by redistribution will have prolonged effects.
> Decreased plasma protein binding (PPB).
> Decreased drug metabolism and excretion.
> Increased drug uptake and distribution due to increased cardiac output, increased alveolar ventilation and increased TBW.

What effect do these pharmacokinetic and pharmacodynamic changes have on the commonly used drugs in anaesthesia?

Inhalational agents:

> Gas inductions are faster due to increased alveolar ventilation compared with FRC, high cardiac output, lower blood/gas solubility and lower tissue/blood solubility of volatile agents.
> MAC is age related. MAC values for an infant are:
> • sevoflurane = 3.3%
> • isoflurane = 1.9%
> • desflurane = 9.4%.

Barbiturates:

> Increased sensitivity to thiopentone and a more prolonged recovery (due to reduced V_d and redistribution).

Propofol:
> Licensed for induction in infants over 1 month and for infusion in children aged 3 years and above.
> Painful on injection (it is acceptable to add a small amount of 1% lignocaine to the propofol).

Opioids:
> Increased sensitivity due to reduced PPB, reduced hepatic metabolism and immature blood–brain barrier.
> Beware of using narcotics and sedative agents in preterm babies and neonates due to the increased risk of apnoea.

Muscle relaxants:
> Depolarising – decreased sensitivity to suxamethonium due to increased V_d and immature neuromuscular junction; therefore, higher dose used (2 mg/kg).
> Non-depolarising – atracurium has increased V_d but also increased clearance and so very little change in overall pharmacokinetics.

Local anaesthetics:
> Decreased protein binding and reduced metabolism increase risk of toxicity.

Intraosseous route (IO):
> In emergency setting, when intravenous access cannot be gained, intraosseous access can be life saving.
> In the long bones, the medullary cavity consists of a network of venous sinusoids that drain into large medullary venous channels. These in turn drain into nutrient or emissary vessels. These vessels exit the bone via the nutrient foramina and empty directly into the systemic venous circulation.
> All resuscitation fluids, drugs and blood products can be administered through the IO route.
> Anatomical landmarks (note that there are other sites that can be used, e.g. sternum):
  • Tibia: medial side, 2–3 cm below the tibial tuberosity
  • Femur – 3 cm above the lateral condyle
    (these sites avoid epiphyseal growth plates and joint spaces)
> Commercially prepared, single-use needles should ideally be used (many now come as powered drill devices).
> Can be left in for up to 72 hours (although the risk of infection increases with time).
> Complications: Infection, extravasation, dislodgement of needle, embolism, compartment syndrome due to extravasation, fracture, pain.
> Contraindications: fracture of target bone, recent IO access (in last 24–48 hours), signs of infection at insertion site, osteogenesis imperfecta.

Table 40.2 Paediatric drug doses

Drug	Dose
Atropine	10–20 mcg/kg
Adrenaline (cardiac arrest) – 1:10 000	10 mcg/kg or 0.1 ml/kg
Suxamethonium	2 mg/kg
Propofol	2–5 mg/kg
Fentanyl	1–3 mcg/kg
Morphine	IV: 50-100 mcg/kg
	PO: 100–200 mcg/kg
Atracurium	0.5 mg/kg
Reversal	Neostigmine: 50 mcg/kg / Glycopyrrolate 10 mcg/kg (easy way to remember is 0.1 ml of premixed ampoule for every 5 kg)
Ondansetron	0.1 mg/kg
Dexamethasone	0.1 mg/kg
Cyclizine	1 mg/kg
Paracetamol	IV: 15 mg/kg if >10 kg (max 90 mg/kg/day)
	IV: 10 mg/kg in neonates and infants <10 kg (max 60 mg/kg/day)
	PO: loading dose: 20 mg/kg; subsequent doses: 15 mg/kg
Diclofenac	1 mg/kg
Ibuprofen (give only for >6 months and >7 kg)	5 mg/kg (max 30 mg/kg/day)

41. PREGNANCY

The changes in maternal physiology are covered in the physiology section (Study Guide 1, Chapter 37). In this question we consider how these changes affect our choice of anaesthetic and why. The following refers to a pregnant patient who is undergoing non-obstetric surgery.

Which general issues should be considered when planning to anaesthetise a pregnant woman?

General anaesthesia during pregnancy is associated with an increased risk of intrauterine growth retardation, early labour and early infant death. For these reasons, elective surgery is contraindicated during pregnancy. If surgery cannot be delayed until after delivery, ideally it should take place in the second trimester.

> Less than 2 weeks' gestation: anaesthesia will have an 'all or nothing effect' on the pregnancy, i.e. it will continue apparently unaffected or will be lost.
> 3–8 weeks' gestation: organogenesis takes place, and anaesthesia is best avoided.
> 8 weeks+: risk of growth retardation with anaesthesia.
> Third trimester: risk of precipitating premature labour is increased.
> Concerns are growing that exposure to anaesthesia may adversely affect neurodevelopment in the developing brain. This may have implications for the fetus, but at the time of publication there is not a great deal of data from this emerging field.

The following factors are of importance:
> There are two patients to consider, though the mother's needs must take priority.
> • The case should be discussed with a senior anaesthetist.
> • Surgery should be carried out by a senior surgeon who can complete the procedure in a timely manner.
> The type of surgery proposed.
> • Consider whether regional anaesthetic techniques would be appropriate.
> The stage of the pregnancy and its effect on maternal physiology (for details *see* answer on 'Pregnancy' in *Study Guide 1*, Chapter 37).
> • Stomach emptying may be delayed from 12 weeks onwards, so do not use a laryngeal mask airway beyond the first trimester; patients should be intubated.
> • The most teratogenic period is thought to be 31–71 days. From 24 weeks onwards, the fetus may potentially survive outside the uterus.
> • The choice of anaesthetic drugs and their potential effects on the fetus must be taken into consideration (*see* list of drug effects at end of this question).

How would you anaesthetise a woman who is 24 weeks pregnant for an appendicectomy?

> **Pre-operatively:**
> - Inform the anaesthetic consultant of the patient.
> - Confirm the diagnosis and the need for the operation with the surgeons.
> - Inform the obstetricians of the plan for surgery and arrange appropriate fetal monitoring (*see* below).
> - Take consent from the woman for rapid sequence induction of general anaesthesia.

> **Induction:**
> - Place the table on a left lateral tilt, to reduce the risk of aorto-caval compression by the gravid uterus (All pregnant patients should be 'tilted' from 20 weeks' gestation onwards)
> - Gain IV access with a large bore (≥16 G) cannula.
> - Have a low threshold for inserting an arterial line, both to monitor BP and to allow regular blood gas analysis.
> - Pre-oxygenate at 30° head up to maintain FRC.
> - Ensure adequate preoxygenation, as pregnant women have a reduced FRC and increased oxygen consumption and consequently desaturate more rapidly. In addition, intubation may be more difficult because of enlarged breasts making insertion of the laryngoscope awkward, so consider using a short-handled laryngoscope.
> - Induction drugs: thiopentone 5 mg/kg and suxamethonium 2 mg/kg.

> **Intra-operative:**
> - Avoid hypoxia or hypercarbia as these will alter blood flow to the placental bed. The fetus can adapt to short periods of maternal hypoxia by increasing its oxygen extraction, but in the face of long-standing hypoxia, the utero-placental bed will constrict and fetal hypoxia will result. Maternal hyperoxia is not detrimental to the fetus but maternal hypercarbia results in fetal respiratory acidosis as the CO_2 passes freely across the placenta.
> - MAC falls in pregnancy, but maintain adequate end-tidal volatile concentration to ensure that the patient is not aware.
> - Maintain relaxation with atracurium, rocuronium or vecuronium, none of which cross the placenta in significant amounts.
> - Provide analgesia with paracetamol and morphine. Do not give NSAIDs in the third trimester as they promote closure of the ductus arteriosus.
> - Give fluid, guided by clinical parameters: BP, heart rate and urine output.
> - If vasopressors are needed, ephedrine has a long history of use in obstetric anaesthesia and is thought to have least effect on the placental blood flow, although phenylephrine and metaraminol are used as first-line therapies in many units.
> - The issue of whether the fetus should be monitored with a CTG intra-operatively is contentious and depends on several factors:

> Monitoring is useful only if it will change management and so if the fetus is unable to survive outside of the uterus (traditionally accepted to be <24 weeks' gestation) there is no useful reason to monitor it intra-operatively.

> If the fetus is viable, there may be an argument to monitor to allow delivery, should it show signs of distress; however, the fetus will also experience the effects of general anaesthesia administered to the mother and so its CTG trace will lose variability and become difficult/impossible to interpret, rendering monitoring useless.

> If monitoring is applied, there must be someone present at all times who can interpret it and make the necessary decisions based on the evidence available.

> As a primary candidate, you should have a grasp of the issues above. In reality, it is sensible for the pregnant woman to have a CTG performed before the operation and after recovery from the anaesthetic to assess the condition of the fetus.

> **Post-operatively:**
>   - Extubate the patient awake and sitting up. Check for an air leak with the cuff deflated to ensure no laryngeal oedema.
>   - Ensure sufficient analgesia; the patient must be able to cough and breathe easily to avoid chest infection, hyperventilation causing a respiratory alkalosis or hypoventilation causing acidosis.
>   - Discharge to an appropriate level of care, depending on patient's condition.

THE EFFECT OF DRUGS ON THE MOTHER AND THE FETUS

At 24 weeks, the fetus is past the 'teratogenic window' (31–71 days). There are few certainties about the use of drugs in pregnancy, and although many anaesthetic agents are thought to be safe from anecdotal evidence, the manufacturers will not officially endorse their use in pregnancy.

NITROUS OXIDE	Inhibits methionine-synthase and tetrahydrofolate reductase and has been shown to be teratogenic in rats. However, this was when used at high concentration for prolonged periods. The clinical implication of this, when used for a short period of time in humans, is questionable, and certainly it provides the mainstay of analgesia during labour.
VOLATILE AGENTS	There are many conflicting studies, some-showing potential teratogenicity in animals, although the design of some of these is questionable. At best, the clinical relevance of these findings is not clear. Most would advocate the use of isoflurane or sevoflurane where necessary.
THIOPENTONE	Teratogenic in high doses in animals. Causes a fall in uteroplacental blood flow (up to 35%), which is not sustained. This is the intravenous induction agent of choice.
PROPOFOL	Does not alter uterine blood flow, but studies show it decreases perinatal survival and so the manufacturers advise against using in pregnancy. Despite this, it is used as the first line induction agent for pregnant women in many centres because of its familiarity amongst anaesthetists along with the decline in the use of thiopentone. This trend is likely to continue, especially in light of the finding of NAP 5, which showed a higher incidence of accidental awareness in pregnant women undergoing Caesarean section under GA (1:670) using thiopentone.
NON-DEPOLARISING MUSCLE RELAXANTS	Non-teratogenic, and these bulky drugs do not cross the placenta well. Their duration of action may be prolonged, presumably due to altered hepatic metabolism. This is not true of atracurium because of Hoffman degradation.
AMIDE LOCAL ANAESTHETICS	Not teratogenic.
OPIOIDS	Considered safe in pregnancy at appropriate doses.

42. ELDERLY PATIENT

There have been several reports (e.g. NCEPOD's 2010 report on 'Elective and Emergency Surgery in the Elderly') that have highlighted that elderly patients are receiving substandard peri-operative care, which is resulting in increased morbidity and mortality. In response to this, the AAGBI updated their guidelines on the 'Peri-operative Care of the Elderly' in 2014, and this chapter highlights the key recommendations. The pathophysiology of ageing is covered in Study Guide 1, *Chapter 40.*

What are the anaesthetic considerations for the elderly patient?

Elderly patients are not a homogenous group and age, per se, cannot be used as a sole indicator of peri-operative risk. It is possible for a 20-year-old to have more significant co-morbidities than a 90-year-old and present with a higher peri-operative risk. However, elderly patients are often complex due to a combination of age-related physiological decline, co-morbidities, cognitive impairment, frailty and polypharmacy. This is associated with an increased risk of morbidity and mortality after elective and especially emergency surgery. Therefore, good peri-operative care is essential in reducing this risk and improving outcome.

General principles:
> Multidisciplinary care improves outcome for elderly surgical patients and the anaesthetist is an integral part of the multidisciplinary team (MDT).
> Decision to operate should be made at consultant level in conjunction with the patient, family and MDT.
> Appropriately experienced senior personnel should be available to anaesthetise and operate on the patient.
> Suitable level of post-operative care should be arranged (e.g. HDU or ITU).

Pre-operative assessment:
> A detailed medical and anaesthetic history is important, but this can sometimes be difficult due to deafness, aphasia and cognitive impairment or dementia.
> Some patients are poor historians and may not be aware of their medical issues or medication.
> A collaborative history from family members or carers can be useful.

History:

> Background to admission – e.g. if patient had a fall and sustained a fractured neck of femur, it is essential to identify whether the fall was mechanical or secondary to another cause, like syncope.
> Co-morbidities should be identified along with their severity.
> Pacemakers (PPMs) and implantable defibrillators (ICDs) need to be identified – ICDs need to be turned off prior to surgery and PPMs should have been checked within the last 6 months – liaise early with pacemaker clinic. Consideration needs to be made on the choice of intra-operative diathermy (*see Study Guide 1*, Chapter 61, 'Diathermy').
> Gastro-oesophageal reflux disease (GORD) is more common – this can increase the risk of aspiration.
> Joint replacements are more common – this affects placement of the diathermy pad and can affect patient positioning for surgery.
> Drug history and allergies – polypharmacy is common and there is increased risk of drug interactions.
> Functional capacity – premorbid level of exercise tolerance (e.g. ability to walk on flat for a specified distance, ability to climb a flight of stairs without stopping, ability to perform activities of daily living independently) provides an indication of cardiopulmonary reserve. It is important to identify where necessary what the limiting factor to exercise tolerance is (e.g. arthritic hip pain, calf claudication pain, chest pain, shortness of breath, balance, fragility).
> Social circumstances – knowledge of this (e.g. nursing home, social care package) helps discharge planning.
> Drug chart and medical note review.
> Nutritional assessment – all elderly patients should have a nutritional assessment on admission. Good nutrition facilitates healing and recovery. If malnutrition is identified, oral nutritional supplements (e.g. iron, vitamin B_{12}, folate) should be commenced. In some cases, nasogastric feeding may be required.

Examination:

> Mini Mental State score – this is useful to identify early onset dementia and memory impairment. It provides a benchmark that can be referred to in the post-operative period.
> Targeted examination should be performed – previously unrecognised pathology may be identified (e.g. ejection systolic murmur of aortic stenosis).
> Observation chart review – baseline blood pressure should be noted, as patients are prone to intra-operative hypotension.

Investigations:

> ECG, FBC, U&Es, blood sugar – minimum data set required.
> Targeted investigations as required – e.g. cardiac ECHO if murmur or heart failure suspected, CXR if lower respiratory tract infection or heart failure is suspected.

Intra-operative considerations:

The choice of anaesthesia; regional or general has not been shown to have any significant difference in patient outcome. What is more important is that the technique used must be administered responsively taking into account the patient's physiological status.

> **Level of monitoring:**
> • Low threshold for invasive blood pressure monitoring in cases where large blood loss or fluid shifts are expected and/or an underlying cardiovascular disease is suspected.
> • Depth of anaesthesia monitoring (e.g. BIS or entropy) – this is useful as the dose of anaesthetic agents required to induce and maintain anaesthesia decreases with increasing age, but the deleterious cardiovascular effects of these agents increase. Monitoring depth of anaesthesia helps titrate dose to effect, minimising hypotension and overdose.
> **Drugs:**
> • Increased sensitivity to induction agents, inhalational agents, benzodiazepines and opioids – increased risk of hypotension and effects of these drugs are more prolonged – reduced doses should be used.
> • Arm–brain circulation is increased – intravenous induction agents should be administered slowly and at a reduced dose.
> • Autonomic responses are blunted – patients are more prone to hypotension.
> **Intravenous access:**
> • Veins are more mobile.
> • Cannulas are more prone to tissuing.
> • Skin is more prone to damage on removal of cannula dressings.
> **Airway:**
> • Pre-oxygenate all patients as age causes a gradual increase in closing capacity, increasing risk of desaturation.
> • Edentulous patients are more difficult to face-mask ventilate.
> • Neck stiffness, cervical spondylosis or arthritis may limit neck extension, making airway maintenance and intubation more difficult.
> • GORD increases risk of aspiration.

> Patient positioning – meticulous care to protect pressure points with adequate padding is essential as risk of neuropraxia and pressure sores is increased.
> Warming – patients are prone to hypothermia so fluid warmers and body warmers should be routinely used and intra-operative temperature monitoring be undertaken.
> Maintenance – MAC is reduced in elderly. Short-acting agents (e.g. desflurane and sevoflurane) are preferred.
> Fluid management – fluid and electrolyte therapy can be challenging in elderly patients due to reduced homeostatic compensation for blood and/or fluid loss (in addition, patients may be taking diuretics). Hydration status should be based on pre-operative hydration, intra-operative losses, urine output, blood pressure and cardiac output monitoring parameters when applicable. Patients are prone to both dehydration (if nil by mouth times have been excessive) and fluid overload especially if cardiac failure or renal failure is present. Aim to maintain euvolaemia.

Post-operative considerations:

> **Analgesia:**
> - Inadequate analgesia for elderly surgical patients contributes to post-operative morbidity including delirium, cardiorespiratory complications (pain increases sympathetic drive, which increases myocardial oxygen consumption) and failure to mobilise.
> - Pain should be assessed regularly and pain levels and sedation scores documented.
> - Assessment can be difficult due to cognitive impairment, dementia and aphasia, and therefore non-verbal cues (e.g. facial expression, posture, grimacing) should also be used.
> - The use of peri-operative analgesia protocols improves patient satisfaction but should be individualised for each patient (e.g. previous chronic pain status, renal function).
> - A multimodal approach to analgesia is best (e.g. local anaesthetic infiltration by surgeons, wound catheters, regional anaesthetic techniques and WHO analgesic ladder).
> - NSAIDs should be used with caution at the lowest dose and for the shortest duration due to the risk of gastric bleeding and nephrotoxicity. Proton pump inhibitors should be prescribed and U&Es be monitored.
> - Morphine and other opiates are effective but should be administered cautiously and dose adjusted, especially in patients with renal impairment, respiratory compromise or cognitive impairment.
> - Acute pain team should be involved.

> **Post-operative delerium:**
> - Some decline in post-operative cognitive function is common in elderly patients. Delirium in the recovery room is a strong predictor for post-operative delerium.
> - Features include acute confusion, disorientation, restlessness, agitation, fear, disturbed sleep, and hallucinations with symptoms often being worse at night.
> - Causes include drugs (e.g. atropine, benzodiazepines, opioids, antihistamines, sedative hypnotics and corticosteroids), infection (e.g. UTI), metabolic (e.g. hypo/hypernatraemia), hypoperfusion (e.g. blood loss or low cardiac output state), hypoxia/hypercarbia and pain.
> - High-quality peri-operative care reduces the incidence of delirium.

> **Post-operative cognitive dysfunction (POCD):**
> - Resembles dementia and can present weeks or months after surgery.
> - Features include change in mood and behaviour, impairment in memory, learning, language and motor function.
> - Diagnosis requires formal neuropsychological testing.
> - Up to 25% of elderly patients can be affected at 1 week post-operatively and 10% at 3 months.
> - Treatment involves good analgesia and correction of physiological parameters, and involvement of psychogeriatricians.

> **Re-enablement:**

Early mobilisation, rehabilitation, physiotherapy and occupational therapy facilitate good post-operative outcome. 'Re-enablement' is the process of getting a patient to return to their pre-operative functional level and involves an MDT approach at each stage of the patient's journey; from their admission, operation, post-operative care and rehabilitation. In order to have a good outcome, the patient must receive a high standard of care at each phase of their care pathway. The anaesthetist plays a vital role in risk stratification, ensuring age-appropriate anaesthesia, fluid therapy, thermoregulation, analgesia, communication and arranging the appropriate level of post-operative care.

43. DOWN'S SYNDROME

Down's syndrome (DS) is one of the most common chromosomal abnormalities, occurring in approximately 1 in 700 live births. It is due to the presence of either a whole or part of an extra 21st chromosome and is hence termed trisomy 21. In the majority of these cases the cause is non-disjunction of the chromosomes (95%) but it can also be due to translocation.

What are the anaesthetic considerations in a patient with Down's syndrome?

Patients with DS may have several anatomical and physiological abnormalities that can cause problems during anaesthesia. Consequently, these cases should be discussed with a consultant anaesthetist. The anaesthetic considerations are best described in terms of organ systems.

> **Nervous system:**
>   • Learning difficulties may lead to an anxious and uncooperative patient. Try to establish a rapport with the patient, tailor your explanation of the anaesthetic to their level of understanding and consider pre-medicating with an anxiolytic or sedative agent.
> **Respiratory system:**
>   • Atlanto-axial and atlanto-occipital instability, which is partly due to ligament laxity and can lead to spinal cord compression. Great care must be taken when positioning the head during intubation. Ask pre-operatively about symptoms of spinal cord compression (numbness and tingling of the arms and fingers) and consider requesting flexion-extension views of the C-spine.
>   • Micrognathia, small mouth, macroglossia, and short neck may all contribute to difficulties during intubation and therefore these must be anticipated. A difficult airway trolley with appropriate emergency drugs should be ready and available. In reality, increased ligament laxity usually means that intubation is not difficult.
>   • Excessive salivation can obscure the view during laryngoscopy and can be an aspiration risk. Consider pre-medicating with an anti-sialogogue.
>   • Adeno-tonsillar hypertrophy and oro-pharyngeal hypotonia may lead to obstructive sleep apnoea. Elicit features of this condition during the pre-operative assessment (snoring, daytime somnolence, ECG evidence of right heart strain). Upper airway obstruction can worsen after anaesthesia and opioids so consider extended recovery or HDU environment in the post-operative period.
>   • Subglottic and tracheal stenosis – consider using a smaller than predicted endotracheal tube.

> **Cardiovascular system:**
  - Congenital heart disease occurs in up to 50% of patients with DS and common abnormalities include ASD, VSD, PDA and TOF. Apart from TOF, all of these defects cause a left-to-right shunt, which can ultimately lead to pulmonary hypertension. Full review of the medical notes with a thorough history and examination is essential. If congenital heart disease is suspected, patients must be investigated and optimised by a cardiologist prior to surgery. Consider the need for prophylactic antibiotics at induction to prevent endocarditis.
  - Difficult venipuncture – this can be due to obesity and/or learning difficulties. Consider pre-medicating patients with topical local anaesthetic agents applied to potential venipuncture sites.
> **Gastrointestinal system:**
  - Gastro-oesophageal reflux, duodenal atresia and gastric paresis occur with increased frequency and all increase the risk of aspiration during induction of anaesthesia. Therefore, consider early NGT placement, pre-medicating with prokinetic agents and antacids and/or a rapid sequence induction technique.
> **General:**
  - Obesity
  - Increased incidence of hypothyroidism
  - Impaired immunity
  - Increased incidence of leukaemia
  - Increased incidence of hepatitis B

44. SICKLE CELL ANAEMIA

What is sickle cell anaemia?

Sickle cell anaemia, or disease, is a haemoglobinopathy with autosomal recessive inheritance. It occurs because of a point mutation on the gene coding for normal haemoglobin (HbA) on chromosome 11, which causes the substitution of valine for glutamic acid at position 6 on the β-haemoglobin chain. This results in the formation of an abnormal β-haemoglobin chain, referred to as 'HbS'.

Homozygotes (HbSS) have only abnormal haemoglobin. Heterozygotes (HbAS) are said to have 'sickle cell trait', and possess both abnormal and normal haemoglobin. The trait is carried by 25% of West Africans, 10% of African Americans and also by those of East Indian, Middle Eastern and Mediterranean origin, where selective pressures of malaria have driven its inheritance. Sickle cell trait is thought to confer some protection against falciparum malaria as the parasite normally completes part of its life cycle within red blood cells. The lifespan of the red blood cells carrying HbS is reduced, and this prevents the parasite from completing its life cycle.

What do you understand by the term 'sickling'?

At low partial pressures of oxygen, deoxygenated HbS polymerises, becomes insoluble and precipitates to form elongated crystals or 'tactoids'. These cause the red blood cell to become rigid and form a 'sickle' shape.

This process increases in the presence of hypoxia, acidosis, dehydration and hypothermia. The degree of sickling is proportional to the concentration of the abnormal haemoglobin, HbS, present in the blood.

In homozygotes, HbS polymerises at PaO_2s between 5 and $6\,kP_a$, and so the red blood cells of these patients sickle continuously within the venous circulation.

In heterozygotes with only 20–45% of abnormal haemoglobin, sickling occurs at much lower PaO_2 of 2–$3\,kP_a$.

Sickled blood cells increase blood viscosity, reduce flow and occlude smaller capillaries causing venous thrombosis and distal organ infarcts. They have a reduced lifespan of 10–20 days, compared to the normal lifespan of 120 days. Consequently, sickle cell disease sufferers are typically anaemic (haemolytic) and jaundiced. HbS shifts the oxyhaemoglobin dissociation curve to the right.

What are the complications associated with sickle cell disease?

Patients with sickle cell trait are usually asymptomatic under normal conditions. Those with sickle cell disease can suffer multi-organ pathology associated with a life expectancy of 40–50 years. Clinical features in those with sickle cell disease only appear from 6 months of age as adult haemoglobin begins to replace fetal, which has no β chains. Homozygotes suffer periods where their disease is worse, called 'sickle cell crises'.

Sickle cell crises:

> **Vaso-occlusive:** Sickled cells obstruct blood flow to an organ or tissue. Most patients have infarcted their spleens by an early age and are on lifelong prophylactic penicillin. Pain control is with simple analgesia and opiates.

> **Sequestration:** Painful splenic enlargement results in anaemia and abdominal distension. Management is supportive.

> **Aplastic:** Usually triggered by infection with parvovirus B19, which arrests red cell production for 2–3 days. Reticulocyte count and Hb fall acutely. In normal individuals this is not clinically significant, but in sickle cell homozygotes who already have shortened red cell survival, it can result in life-threatening anaemia.

> **Haemolytic:** The rate of red cell breakdown increases. This is rare and usually seen in only those with co-existing G6PD deficiency.

Systemic complications:

> **Haematological:**
  - Chronic haemolytic anaemia
  - Crises, as above

> **Respiratory:**
  - Acute chest syndrome, which manifests as pleuritic pain, cough, dyspnoea, haemoptysis and fever. Recurrent episodes can lead to pulmonary hypertension and chronic respiratory failure

> **Cardiovascular:**
  - Hypertension and left ventricular hypertrophy

> **Gastrointestinal:**
  - Acute sequestration syndrome of red blood cells in the liver or spleen
  - Haemosiderosis, secondary to repeated transfusions
  - Gallstones, secondary to chronic haemolysis

> **Genitourinary:**
  - Haematuria
  - Renal failure secondary to acute papillary necrosis
  - Priapism

> **Neurological complications:**
  - Stroke
  - Meningitis

> **Immune system:**
  - Splenic infarction increases the risk of infection by encapsulated organisms including *Streptococcus pneumoniae*, *Haemophilus influenzae* and *Neisseria meningitidis*. Asplenic patients must be vaccinated against these organisms and take oral penicillin daily

> **Eyes:**
  - Proliferative retinopathy

> **Musculoskeletal:**
  - Deformity of skull and long bones secondary to compensatory hyperplasia
  - Bone pain
  - Osteomyelitis, commonly caused by *Salmonella*
  - Avascular necrosis, most commonly affects hip joint, but other major joints may be involved

> **Skin:**
  - Ulceration

> **Chronic pain:**
  - Opioid tolerance
  - Pain management issues

Which investigations would help confirm a diagnosis of sickle cell anaemia?

> **FBC:**
>   - ↓ Hb (6–8 g/dL)
>   - Reticulocyte count (10–20%)
> **LFTs:**
>   - Bilirubin
> **Blood film:**
>   - Target cells
>   - Sickled cells
>   - Howell–Jolly bodies
> **Sickledex test:**
>   - Sickling is induced by the addition of sodium metabisulfite to the sample.
>   - This confirms only the presence of HbS but cannot differentiate between HbAS and HBSS so is only a screening test.
> **Electrophoresis** (definitive test)
>   - Determines the type and proportion of HbS present and is therefore diagnostic

How would you prepare for and administer an anaesthetic to a patient with sickle cell disease?

> **Pre-operative:**
>   - Involve the haematology team.
>   - Assess disease severity by assessing clinical features and laboratory findings.
>   - For major elective intra-cavity surgery, aim for an HbS concentration of <40% and an Hb of 10–12 g/dL. This may be achieved by exchange transfusion.
>   - Cross-match blood early, as antibodies can be generated in response to previous transfusions. Consequently, the process of cross-matching maybe prolonged and it can take up to 48 hours to source suitable blood when unusual antibodies are present.
>   - Ensure the patient is fully vaccinated and on regular penicillin and folic acid.
>   - Keep nil by mouth for the minimum possible duration and prescribe intravenous fluids during this time.
>   - Avoid sedatives as this can cause hypoventilation leading to respiratory acidosis and hypoxia.
> **Peri-operative:** Standard anaesthetic techniques may be used but particular attention must be paid to the potential problems of hypoxia, hypothermia, acidosis, dehydration and pain.
>   - **Oxygenation:** Pre-oxygenate patients well and maintain oxygenation with an appropriate FiO_2.
>   - **Normothermia:** Use fluid warmers and warming blankets throughout the procedure and minimise shivering as this consumes a vast amount of oxygen.
>   - **Avoid circulatory stasis:** Position the patient well to prevent blood stasis in dependent parts or limbs. Avoid the use of arterial tourniquets: although not absolutely contraindicated, they should be used with extreme caution. Maintain good cardiac output to prevent venous sludging. Ideally, vasopressors should be avoided.
>   - **Hydration:** Give intravenous fluids to maintain hydration and prevent venous sludging.
>   - **Avoid acidosis:** Ventilate to normocapnia to prevent respiratory acidosis.
>   - **Analgesia:** Maintain good analgesia as this reduces catecholamine surges and minimises oxygen consumption. Be aware that these patients may be opioid tolerant and therefore are likely to benefit from early review by the pain management team.
>   - **Intravenous regional anaesthesia** (e.g. Bier's block): Such techniques are absolutely contraindicated in sickle cell disease, because the prolonged venous stasis would result in sickling through the limb.

> **Post-operative:** Vigilance to avoid precipitating a crisis must continue into the post-operative period for both homo- and heterozygous patients.
  - Homozygotes are not suitable candidates for day surgery and those undergoing intermediate to high-risk procedures should be considered for critical care post-operatively.
  - Administer supplemental oxygen.
  - Continue intravenous fluids until patient is eating and drinking.
  - Ensure effective analgesia using a multimodal approach and involve the pain team.
  - Avoid hypothermia.

45. RHEUMATOID ARTHRITIS

What special considerations should be made when anaesthetising a patient with rheumatoid arthritis?

Rheumatoid arthritis (RA) is a multi-system disease which causes a symmetrical deforming inflammatory polyarthropathy. It is more common in women than men and affects approximately 2% of the population worldwide. Its extra-articular features are extensive and some are of particular importance to us as anaesthetists. It is easiest to consider the effects of the disease in systems and consequences of medication.

General:
> Patients are often frail and suffer chronic pain.
> Steroid therapy causes thinning of the skin and care must be taken when moving patients or when removing sticky tape as this can tear fragile skin.
> Patients must be carefully positioned on the operating table. Ideally, they should position themselves on the table prior to the induction of anaesthesia. Pressure areas must be closely monitored.
> If planning a regional block, ensure the patient is able to position themselves to allow for this.
> Stiffness, deformity, joint pain and lack of fine motor control may render patients unable to use devices such as patient-controlled analgesia pumps.

> **Musculoskeletal:**
  • Temporomandibular joint involvement may limit mouth opening.
  • Atlanto-axial subluxation (most commonly anterior subluxation) occurs in up to 25% of RA patients and may be asymptomatic. Search for signs in the history, e.g. tingling or weakness in the limbs or loss of fine motor control. Assess the patient's range of neck movement and ensure no movement outside this range once they are anaesthetised. If there is any doubt about neck stability, cervical spine X-rays (flexion, extension and peg views) may help. A gap of >3 mm between the odontoid peg and the arch of the atlas in lateral flexion suggests the risk of anterior subluxation. An unstable neck may need to be surgically stabilised prior to other elective surgery. If there is actual or potential subluxation, use manual in-line stabilisation when manipulating the airway and have a low threshold to use awake fibre-optic intubation.
  • Crico-arytenoid involvement can cause hoarseness and limit airflow, causing stridor in severe cases. If this is a concern, request a pre-operative nasendoscopic assessment of the larynx by the ENT surgeons.

> **Cardiovascular:**
>   - Pericardial effusions are uncommon and usually asymptomatic. They can rarely cause tamponade.
>   - Valvular or myocardial involvement is rare. Request a transthoracic echocardiogram if complications are suspected.
> **Respiratory:**
>   - Pleural effusions are the most common lung manifestation of the disease.
>   - Rheumatoid nodules may be up to 3cm in diameter and can be mistaken for carcinoma.
>   - Lung fibrosis is a rare complication and may be caused by the disease or by treatment with methotrexate. If respiratory abnormalities are found, consider lung function testing.
> **Renal:**
>   - RA can cause amyloidosis, which can lead to renal failure.
>   - Drugs may affect the kidneys but analgesic nephropathy is rare nowadays.
> **Nervous system:**
>   - Carpel tunnel syndrome can occur.
>   - Polyneuropathy is a rare manifestation.
>   - Compression of nerves at the cord or root may occur, so careful positioning is important.
> **Haematology:**
>   - Anaemia of chronic disease
>   - Anaemia secondary to gastrointestinal blood loss caused by NSAID use.
> **Eyes:**
>   - Keratoconjunctivitis sicca (i.e. dry eyes).

Drugs:
> **Steroids:** Patients on steroid therapy may need steroid supplementation in the peri-operative period.
> **NSAIDs:** Check a baseline renal function and, unless contraindicated, continue with NSAIDs in the post-operative period to help mobilisation.
> **Disease modifying anti-rheumatic drugs (DMARDs):** e.g. gold, penicillamine, and methotrexate. These can all cause immuno-suppression, which may delay wound healing and increase the risk of infection. Do not stop these drugs without discussion with the patient's rheumatologist as their benefits may outweigh their risks.

Post-operative care:
> Continue rheumatoid medication if possible.
> Keep patients well hydrated and monitor renal function.
> Give early and regular physiotherapy, aiming for rapid return to baseline mobility.
> While immobile, patients will need DVT prophylaxis.

ATLANTO- AXIAL SUBLUXATION

What does 'atlanto-axial subluxation' actually mean?

The Atlas is another name for the first cervical vertebra (C1). It is derived from Greek mythology, as the 'Atlas' holds up the 'globe' that is the skull. The Atlas is unique in that it has no body; instead it is fused to that of C2 below it. C2 is known as 'the Axis'. The name 'Axis' comes from the Latin, meaning 'axle'. It is so called because it forms a pivot on which C1, which carries the head, can rotate. The odontoid peg, or dens, is a protrusion from the upper anterior surface of C2 which sticks up through where the body of C1 should be to articulate with the anterior arch of C1. This is a non-weight-bearing joint and its unique structure allows the wide range of movement of the head on the spine.

Subluxation of any joint means partial or incomplete dislocation of that joint. In this situation, the vertebrae of C1 and 2 move out of their correct positions relative to each other and therefore can impinge on the spinal cord. Obviously, cord compression at this high level can be catastrophic. Atlanto-axial subluxation occurs with increased frequency in RA because the disease causes degeneration of the bursa lying next to the transverse ligament of the atlas, causing it to weaken (this is a thick, strap-like ligament which is attached to each side of the anterior arch of the atlas and loops behind the odontoid peg, holding it snugly against the arch). If this ligament becomes lax, the peg is able to move away from the anterior arch of the atlas and to move posteriorly when the neck flexes. As it does this there is a risk that it will impinge on the spinal cord. Although atlanto-axial subluxation is reasonably common on X-ray, symptoms are actually rare.

46. DIABETES

What is diabetes and how is it classified?

Diabetes mellitus (DM) is a group of metabolic diseases characterised by hyperglycaemia and resulting from defects in insulin secretion, insulin action or both. Patients with any form of diabetes may require insulin treatment at some stage of their disease. It can be classified, based on aetiology, as follows:

> **Type 1 diabetes** (previously insulin-dependent diabetes mellitus) Characterised by loss of insulin-producing beta cells of the islets of Langerhans in the pancreas, via an immune or idiopathic mechanism. It usually presents in childhood and requires exogenous insulin administration to prevent ketosis.
> **Type 2 diabetes** (previously non-insulin-dependent diabetes mellitus) Characterised by insulin resistance, which may be combined with relatively reduced insulin secretion. The main risk factors include central obesity, increasing age and family history. Treatment involves increasing physical activity, reducing carbohydrate intake and weight reduction, and may require oral hypoglycaemic agents and/or non-insulin injectables. In later stages, insulin may also be necessary.

Other specific types include:
> Gestational diabetes – any degree of glucose intolerance with onset or first recognition during pregnancy.
> Genetic defects of beta-cell function (e.g. maturity onset diabetes of the young or MODY).
> Genetic defects in insulin action (defects in insulin receptor or post-receptor signal transduction pathways).
> Diseases of the exocrine pancreas (pancreatitis, trauma, infection, pancreatectomy, adenocarcinoma, cystic fibrosis, haemochromatosis).
> Endocrinopathies (acromegaly, Cushing's, glucagonoma, phaeochromocytoma, i.e. increase in hormones that antagonise insulin).
> Drug- or chemical-induced (drugs or toxins that may precipitate diabetes in individuals with insulin resistance, e.g. β-blockers, thiazides, glucocorticoids).
> Infections (congenital rubella, CMV, coxsackievirus B, mumps).
> Uncommon forms of immune-mediated diabetes (anti-insulin receptor antibodies).
> Other genetic syndromes sometimes associated with diabetes (Down's, Klinefelter's, Turner's).

What do you understand by the terms impaired glucose tolerance (IGT) and impaired fasting glucose (IFG)?

Intermediate group of patients whose glucose levels do not meet the criteria for diabetes, but are nevertheless too high to be considered normal. They are considered as having 'pre-diabetes' indicating a relatively high risk of developing DM later. Criteria are:

> IFG: fasting plasma glucose = 5.6–6.9 mmol/L
> IGT: glucose = 7.8–11.1 mmol/L (2-h post glucose load)

What are the complications of diabetes?

> **Acute complications:**
> - Diabetic ketoacidosis (DKA); more common in Type 1 than Type 2.
> - Hyperosmolar non-ketotic state (HONK); more common in Type 2 than Type 1.
> - Hypoglycaemia, usually iatrogenic resulting from excess insulin administration.
>
> All of the acute complications are potentially life-threatening and constitute medical emergencies.

> **Chronic complications:**
> - Vascular – accelerated atherosclerosis, cerebrovascular disease, coronary artery disease, hypertension and peripheral vascular disease.
> - Diabetic nephropathy – early signs of renal failure are proteinuria and elevated serum creatinine.
> - Autonomic neuropathy – postural hypotension and impaired gastric motility.
> - Peripheral neuropathy – increased risk of tissue damage and ulceration.
> - Diabetic retinopathy.
> - Infection – increased risk of post-operative wound infection.
> - Musculoskeletal – collagen glycosylation may lead to stiff joint syndrome and has been associated with a higher incidence of difficult intubation as it can affect the temporomandibular joints.

What are the anaesthetic implications of a diabetic patient presenting for surgery?

The aims of pre-operative assessment are to:
> Determine the severity of any systemic complications.
> Assess the adequacy of blood glucose control.
> Exclude the presence of ketoacidosis.

Diabetic patients are at increased risk of peri-operative complications including silent MI, stroke, pressure sores, infections of wounds/chest/urinary tract, and ketogenesis.

What peri-operative management consideration should be made for patients with Types 1 and 2 diabetes on elective lists?

There is evidence that poor pre-operative glycaemic control is associated with greater post-operative mortality and morbidity after elective surgery, including silent MI, stroke, pressure sores, infections of wounds/chest/urinary tract and ketogenesis.

Peri-operative considerations:
> The patient will undergo a period of enforced fasting – blood glucose will need to be maintained during this period.
> Patients presenting for emergency surgery may be metabolically deranged, with major acid–base and electrolyte disturbances, which need correcting.
> Patients presenting for elective surgery should have good glycaemic control. Measure glycosylated haemoglobin (HbA_{1c}) levels, which correlate with blood glucose control in the preceding 2 months (normal <7%).
> The surgical stress response will cause a rise in blood glucose intra-operatively.
> The patient may not be allowed oral intake of fluid or nutrition for a period post-operatively, e.g. following abdominal laparotomy.

Peri-operative management:
Guidelines were published by NHS Diabetes and the Joint British Diabetes Societies Inpatient Care Group in April 2011 to improve the standard of care received by diabetic patients undergoing elective surgery (some principles can be applied to the emergency setting).

The main recommendations are:

> Minimise starvation time by prioritising diabetic patients on the operating list.
> When starvation times are limited to one meal:
> • patients on oral hypoglycaemic agents should continue only metformin and pioglitazone as normal on the day of surgery and omit all others.
> • patients on insulin should continue intermediate or long-acting insulins and either halve or omit short-acting insulins (this depends on the type of insulin regimen).
> When starvation times are expected to exceed more:
> • all patients should receive a Variable Rate Intravenous Insulin Infusion (VRIII), formerly called insulin sliding scale.
> Measure blood glucose on admission and then hourly intra-operatively and in the immediate post-operative period.
> If pre-operative glucose is above 12 mmol/L, check blood and urinary ketones. If <3+ administer subcutaneous insulin (as per guideline) and reassess; if >3+, then cancel surgery and treat as DKA.
> Implement the WHO Surgical Safety Checklist bundle. The target blood glucose should be 6–10 mmol/L (acceptable range 4–12 mmol/L).
> Use multimodal analgesia and anti-emetics to enable early resumption of usual diet and self-managed diabetes regimen.
> Implement principles of the Enhanced Recovery Programme: early mobilisation with resumption of normal diet and return to usual diabetes management.
> Involve diabetes specialists where indicated.

How is a variable rate intravenous insulin infusion used?

> VRIII are indicated if starvation time is expected to be more than one meal, or if diabetes is decompensated.
> Insulin should be administered via a syringe driver, and intravenous fluid via a volumetric infusion pump, both through a single cannula with one-way or antisiphon valves.
> The recommended intravenous fluid for a VRIII is 0.45% sodium chloride with 5% glucose and either 0.15% potassium chloride (KCl) or 0.3% KCl.
> The dose requires adjusting according to hourly capillary blood glucose (CBG).
> • If CBG is <4 mmol/L reduce VRIII to 0.5 mL/h and administer 10% dextrose (this is to limit ketogenesis that occurs in the absence of background insulin). Stop the infusion only if a long-acting insulin has been continued.
> • Once patient is eating and drinking revert back to their regular medication. Dose adjustments (especially short-acting insulin and sulphonylureas) may be necessary and there should be a period of overlap between VRIII and subcutaneous insulin administration.
> Insulin should be prescribed according to National Patient Safety Agency (NPSA) recommendations for safe use of insulin.

47. HYPERTENSIVE PATIENT

What are the causes of hypertension?

Hypertension can be defined as a systolic blood pressure (SBP) >140mmHg or a diastolic blood pressure (DBP) >90mmHg.

Hypertension is the most common chronic disease in British primary care and almost 50% of people over the age of 65 years have hypertension. Examiners will expect a good understanding of the pathophysiology of the disorder, its anaesthetic implications and its peri-operative management.

Studies have shown that untreated hypertensive patients are at significantly increased risk of stroke, myocardial infarction, heart failure, renal failure and hypertensive retinopathy.

> Primary (essential) hypertension – accounts for 90% of cases
> Secondary hypertension – accounts for 10% of cases. Secondary causes of hypertension:
  - Renal disease (e.g. renal artery stenosis)
  - Endocrine disease (e.g. Conn's syndrome/phaeochromocytoma)
  - Pregnancy-related disease (e.g. pre-eclampsia).

How can hypertension be classified?

Table 47.1 Classification of hypertension

Hypertension	Systolic pressure	Diastolic pressure
- Stage 1 (mild)	140–159	90–99
- Stage 2 (moderate)	160–179	100–109
- Stage 3 (severe)	180–209	110–119
- Stage 4	> 210	> 120
Isolated systolic hypertension	> 150	< 90

What types of medication might a hypertensive patient be taking?

In the primary care setting, basic treatment for primary hypertension may include advice about lifestyle changes such as weight reduction and increased exercise and dietary changes such as reducing salt intake.

The following classes of antihypertensive medication may also be prescribed:

> Diuretics, e.g. bendroflumethiazide
> β-adrenoceptor antagonists, e.g. atenolol
> Angiotensin-converting enzyme inhibitors, e.g. ramipril
> Angiotensin II inhibitors, e.g. losartan
> Calcium channel antagonists, e.g. amlodipine
> α-adrenoceptor antagonists, e.g. doxazosin
> Potassium channel activators, e.g. nicorandil

Discuss the peri-operative management of a hypertensive patient presenting for surgery.

Pre-operative assessment:
> Confirm the diagnosis of hypertension and establish current treatment.
> Confirm the efficacy of treatment, or establish if modification of the antihypertensive regimen is required, e.g. dose alteration, drug class switch or addition.
> If hypertension is severe (i.e. stage 3 – SBP >180 or DBP >110), this should be treated before elective surgery.
> Search for end-organ damage throughout the history, examination and investigations. It is important to establish associated co-morbidity and assess cardio-respiratory performance, e.g. exercise tolerance.
> Investigations may include:
  • ECG (look for left ventricular hypertrophy or strain pattern)
  • Electrolytes (diuretic-induced hypokalaemia or elevated creatinine secondary to ACE inhibitors)

Pre-operative preparation:
> Continue all antihypertensive medications up to and including the morning of surgery except for ACE inhibitors, which should be omitted for 24 hours prior to surgery, as they are associated with severe refractory intra-operative hypotension.

Potential intra-operative problems:
The hypertensive patient is at increased peri-operative risk and the following problems may be encountered intra-operatively:

> Labile blood pressure – lability is more common at certain points such as induction, intubation, start of surgery, extubation and post-operatively if pain is uncontrolled.
> Remember that a hypertrophied left ventricle is at severe risk of peri-operative sub-endocardial myocardial ischaemia. This may occur if there is a fall in coronary perfusion pressure or coronary filling time, and so low BP and tachycardia should be avoided.
> Vasoactive agents should be administered cautiously to hypertensive patients as the response may be exaggerated, particularly if regular antihypertensive medication has been given.
> Organs that autoregulate their blood supply (e.g. cerebral circulation) will have a right shift in the autoregulation curve, which may result in organ blood flow being severely compromised if a hypertensive patient becomes hypotensive.
> Left ventricular diastolic dysfunction is common in hypertensive patients.
> Fluid balance is extremely important, as large fluid shifts are not well tolerated; maintenance of intravascular volume is vital.

Monitoring:
> Invasive blood pressure monitoring with an arterial line should be used for hypertensive patients undergoing major surgery and should be considered on an individual patient basis for other types of surgery.

Post-operatively:
> Rebound hypertension is a common occurrence. Myocardial work is increased by such elevations in blood pressure, but care must be taken not to cause a precipitous fall in blood pressure by rapid administration of further antihypertensives, as this may lead to hypotensive ischaemia.
> A full assessment of the patient in the post-anaesthesia care unit should be performed, looking for potential causes of rebound hypertension (e.g. pain, hypoxia, hypercarbia, fluid overload, hypothermia). Only once these have been dealt with should cautious administration of an antihypertensive be considered.
> Supplemental oxygen should be considered in all hypertensive patients.

When would you cancel a hypertensive patient's operation?

This is not a straightforward question because it requires a risk–benefit analysis, focusing on the urgency of the surgery, the severity of the hypertension and individual patient factors such as the extent and severity of end-organ damage and associated co-morbidities.

There is considerable difference of opinion as to what the threshold blood pressure is for cancelling elective cases in order to optimise treatment. You may, however, be pushed by the examiners to give examples of what types of patient you might cancel, so this list of scenarios may be a sensible guide:

> Severe hypertension (DBP >110 mmHg)/Elective surgery
  • Cancel – treat for at least 1 month prior to reassessment.
> Moderate hypertension (DBP 100–109 mmHg)/End-organ damage/Elective surgery
  • Cancel – treat for at least 1 month prior to reassessment.
> Moderate hypertension (DBP 100–109 mmHg)/No end-organ damage/Elective surgery
  • Cancel – treat for 5–7 days then reassess.
> Mild hypertension (DBP 90–99 mmHg)/Elective surgery
  • Consider peri-operative β-blocker if not contraindicated (e.g. administered 30 minutes prior to surgery) and proceed.

48. CHRONIC OBSTRUCTIVE PULMONARY DISEASE

Chronic obstructive pulmonary disease (COPD) is characterised by an increase in expiratory airflow resistance, which results in:

> *Increased total lung capacity (TLC)*
> *Increased residual volume (RV)*
> *Increased functional residual capacity (FRC)*
> *Reduced forced expiratory volume in 1 second (FEV_1) to FVC ratio (<80%)*

The most important cause of COPD is cigarette smoking and therefore patients with COPD may also suffer from associated smoking-related diseases such as ischaemic heart disease, peripheral vascular disease, cerebrovascular disease and lung cancer.

How would you assess a patient with COPD for anaesthesia?

Assessment is based on taking a relevant history, detailed clinical examination and review of investigations.

History:
> Establish the degree of respiratory compromise, based on:
>   • Exercise tolerance – the ability to climb two flights of stairs without stopping correlates with good cardiorespiratory reserve
>   • Symptoms of dyspnoea – when present at rest or on minimal exertion, this indicates severe compromise
>   • Ability to perform activities of daily living independently
>   • Number of hospital admissions for exacerbations of COPD and their outcome, e.g. admission to ITU
> Establish current treatment regimen, e.g. bronchodilators, steroids, home oxygen.
> Review respiratory physician's clinic letters.
> Obtain a smoking history.

Examination:
> Ability to talk in full sentences
> Peripheral or central cyanosis
> Nicotine-stained fingernails
> Use of accessory respiratory muscles
> Evidence of right heart failure secondary to pulmonary hypertension, e.g. raised jugular venous pressure, hepatomegaly and peripheral oedema
> Chest examination – crackles or wheeze
> Ask to observe the patient walking in the ward, if appropriate

Investigations:

Target investigations to define the extent of the disease, establish pre-operative baseline respiratory function and enable respiratory optimisation.

> Bloods – FBC may reveal polycythaemia from chronic hypoxaemia.
> ECG – may show right ventricular hypertrophy.
> CXR – look for hyperexpanded lung fields or the presence of bullae.
> ABG – on air, as a baseline.
> Pulmonary function tests – spirometry (reduced FEV_1: FVC ratio) and flow–volume loops.
> Indicators of the requirement for likely post-operative ventilation include:
>   • FEV_1 <1 L
>   • FEV_1: FVC ratio <50%
>   • Baseline type 2 respiratory failure

What are the anaesthetic implications for a patient with COPD presenting for surgery?

> Anaesthesia and surgery may result in a peri-operative decline in respiratory function.
> Certain sites of surgery are particularly high risk in terms of post-operative respiratory morbidity in COPD patients, namely thoracic and upper abdominal surgery.
> General anaesthesia results in a reduction in FRC (*see Study Guide 1*, Part 1, Chapter 14, 'Effects of anaesthesia on lung function').
> Atelectasis reduces pulmonary compliance. This may lead to intra-operative and post-operative hypoxaemia and increases the risk of barotrauma in patients requiring ventilation.
> Post-operative hypoventilation is common in patients with COPD, especially when opiate analgesia has been administered.
> Consider the level of care required post-operatively, based on the severity of COPD and the extent of planned surgery. This may range from ward-based care to level 3 ITU support.

How can a patient with COPD be optimised pre-operatively?

A detailed assessment of the patient is essential in order to establish the extent of the disease and so the resulting risk. This allows the employment of targeted interventions to optimise the patient's condition. The following interventions should be made:

> **Smoking cessation** – if smoking is stopped at least 8 weeks prior to surgery, there is a demonstrated reduction in peri-operative respiratory morbidity.
> **Optimal medical treatment of COPD** – a recent review by a respiratory physician is essential to ensure optimal pharmacotherapy, e.g. bronchodilators, steroids and treatment of intercurrent infection.
> **Incentive spirometry** – this has been proven to improve peri-operative outcomes and should be instituted pre-operatively.
> **Peri-operative chest physiotherapy** – to maintain lung volumes, secretion clearance and prevent atelectasis.
> Early post-operative mobilisation.

Regional or general anaesthesia?

This area is controversial as the evidence supporting a reduction in overall peri-operative morbidity and mortality in patients with COPD having surgery under regional anaesthetic techniques is mixed. However, it is clear that excellent post-operative analgesia (via regional techniques or systemic opiates) is essential for good peri-operative outcomes in this patient population.

Certain types of surgery lend themselves extremely well to regional techniques, e.g. orthopaedic lower limb surgery. These operations may be performed under spinal anaesthesia, therefore avoiding the effects of general anaesthesia for the patient with COPD.

Upper abdominal and thoracic surgery also lends itself well to epidural analgesia, allowing excellent post-operative analgesia, which may reduce peri-operative respiratory complications.

49. BURNS AND TRAUMA

How would you assess a patient with burns who presents to A&E?

All burns victims are considered 'trauma patients' and their assessment should follow the Advanced Trauma Life Support (ATLS) guidelines. Assessment and resuscitation must occur simultaneously, with appropriate emergency treatment being instigated as injuries are discovered.

History:
> The ATLS 'AMPLE' history is a useful mnemonic in emergency situations.
  - **A** – Allergies
  - **M** – Medication
  - **P** – Past illnesses/Pregnancy
  - **L** – Last meal
  - **E** – Events related to the injury
> Establish the mechanism of the burn (e.g. explosion: risk of shrapnel and blast injury; enclosed space: risk of inhalational injury; chemical burn: risk to medical team who should wear protective clothing). In children, be aware of the potential for non-accidental injury.
> Ask specifically about other associated injuries (e.g. patient may have jumped out of a window to escape the fire). Head injury, fractures or intra-abdominal injury are not uncommon in this cohort.
> Determine the time of injury, as this will guide fluid resuscitation.

Primary survey:
> **Airway and cervical spine control:**
  - Cervical spine fractures must be suspected so immobilise the patient using either manual in-line immobilisation or three-point fixation technique (hard collar, sand bags and tape).
  - Look for burns to the face, oedema of the lips and oropharynx, singed eyebrows and nasal hair, carbonaceous sputum and drooling. Listen for stridor, wheeze, cough or hoarseness. These features suggest inhalational injury and if present, high-flow, humidified O_2 via face mask with a reservoir bag should be administered.
  - Early endotracheal intubation should be considered as airway oedema can progress rapidly. The endotracheal tube should not be cut shorter due to the risk of ongoing facial oedema.
  - If intubation is needed, call for senior assistance and have the difficult intubation trolley at hand. The patient should remain immobilised during the procedure, unless a life-threatening 'can't intubate, can't ventilate' situation arises, when the airway takes priority over everything else. If time permits and the situation is appropriate, consider an awake fibre-optic intubating technique if there is a high clinical suspicion of an unstable cervical spine fracture.

- Suxamethonium is contraindicated from 6 hours to 2 years after a major burn injury because of the risk of severe hyperkalaemia. There is also an increased resistance to non-depolarising neuromuscular blocking drugs mandating the need for higher doses in these patients. These effects are thought to be due to changes in the volume of drug distribution, up-regulation of nicotinic ACh receptors, sprouting of extra-junctional ACh receptors and alterations in ACh morphology.

> **Breathing:**
- Poisoning due to inhalation of carbon monoxide (CO) (generated by fires in enclosed spaces) and cyanide (generated by burning plastic) is a significant risk.
- Oxygen saturations recorded with a pulse oximeter will be falsely high in the presence of carboxyhaemoglobin (HbCO) and therefore a co-oximeter, which can differentiate HbCO from oxyhaemoglobin, should be used. Arterial blood gas samples should be taken.
- Circumferential burns to the chest can restrict ventilation and an escharotomy may be necessary. These are not usually needed within the first 6 hours of a burn.

> **Circulation and haemorrhage control:**
- Burns are associated with large fluid shifts, as fluid from the intravascular space escapes into the extracellular tissues, causing oedema. Aggressive resuscitation is required to maintain adequate cardiac output and minimise the risk of organ failure.
- Two large-bore 14 G cannula should be sited; this may be difficult if the arms and legs are extensively burned.
- Circumferential burns to limbs can constrict blood supply and may require escharotomies.
- There are several formulae that can be used to calculate the volume for fluid replacement (e.g. Parkland, Mount Vernon and Brook formulae) but the ATLS guidelines recommend the use of the Parkland formula:

> **Parkland formula = 4 mL/kg crystalloid × % burn**
- This is the total volume given over the first 24 hours: half of the total volume should be given over 8 hours, and the remaining half over 16 hours.
- For the second 24 hours, administer fluid at a rate of 2 mL/kg crystalloid × % burn.
- Time is calculated from the time of the burn and not from the time of arrival into hospital.
- This formula only provides an estimate of the fluid volume required for resuscitation. In addition to this, the normal daily fluid requirements must be administered.

> **Neurological assessment and pain control:**
- GCS and pupil reactivity must be assessed as CO poisoning, hypoxia, hypotension or traumatic head injury can impair neurological function.
- Burns may be excruciatingly painful and therefore analgesics, including opiates, should be administered promptly.

> **Burn assessment and avoidance of hypothermia:**
- In an adult, 'Wallace's Rule of Nines' is used to estimate the body surface area (BSA) involved in the burn. The body is divided into anatomical regions that represent 9%, or multiples of 9% of the total body surface; head 9%, arms 9% each, chest and abdomen 18%, back 18% and legs 18% each. The perineum represents 1%.

- The BSA differs in children, where the head represents 18% of the surface area, and the lower limbs a smaller proportion. Paediatric burns charts should be consulted to estimate the extent of the burn.
- The depth of the burn is important in assessing its severity, in wound management and in determining the ultimate cosmetic and functional results. Superficial burns (e.g. sunburn) represent damage to the epidermis. They are erythematous and painful but with no blistering and heal in 2–3 days. Partial thickness burns represent damage to the epidermis and dermis. They are painful, with blisters, and heal in 10 days. Full-thickness burns represent destruction of the epidermis and dermis down to the subcutaneous fat. Hair follicles and pain receptors are lost and so the burns are white, leathery and painless. They heal slowly by wound contracture.
- Patients can become hypothermic rapidly because of impaired homeostasis, heat loss through burns and the resetting of the euthermic temperature to approximately 38.5 °C. This should be minimised by increasing the ambient temperature, covering exposed areas and using fluid warmers and heated blankets.

Secondary survey:
Once the patient is stable, a more detailed clinical assessment should be undertaken.

Investigations:
> **Bloods:**
- FBC may reveal low Hb from blood loss.
- Electrolytes may show hyperkalaemia due to rhabdomyolysis.
- Urea and creatinine may be raised in impending or established renal failure.
> **Cross-match blood:** Patients may need theatre, and blood loss during surgical debridement can be rapid, exceeding 2 mL/kg per 1% of burn treated.
> **Blood gas:**
- CO poisoning causes hypoxia with elevated HbCO levels.
- Cyanide poisoning causes hypoxia with a lactic acidosis and an increased anion gap.
> **ECG:** Arrhythmias can occur due to hyperkalaemia, hypoxia, hypoperfusion or acidosis.
> **Radiological trauma series:** CXR, cervical spine and pelvis.

Which generic management options should be considered in a patient with extensive burns?

Many of these will apply to any sick patient, and a systems-based approach should be used.

> **Analgesia**
> **Gastrointestinal system:**
- Patients become hypercatabolic, requiring an increased daily calorie intake and so nasogastric feeding should be started as soon as possible.
- Ulcer prophylaxis should be given due to the increased risk of Curling's ulcers.
> **Genito-urinary system:**
- A urinary catheter should be inserted and hourly urine output monitored (aiming for at least 0.5 mL/kg/h).
- Renal function must be checked daily as there is a high risk of developing rhabdomyolysis and acute renal failure.
> **Infection:**
- Patients are at increased risk due to loss of the protective skin barrier and generalised immunosuppression.
- Special wound dressings may be used together with topical antimicrobial agents. Prophylactic antibiotics are not used routinely.
- The patient may require tetanus immunisation.

> **Temperature:** Tendency to hypothermia, which can have widespread effects, e.g. inhibits clotting, suppresses the immune system and impair wound healing.
> **Thromboprophylaxis:** Pharmacological (e.g. s/c LMWH) and mechanical thromboprophylaxis if appropriate (e.g. TED stockings +/– pneumatic calf compression).
> **Psychological support:** Patients may require counselling and support to accept both the events causing their injuries and for the resulting disability or change in appearance.
> **Referral to specialist burns centre:** Criteria for transfer include partial or full-thickness burns greater than 10% of BSA in extremes of ages (less than 10 years or older than 50 years), partial or full-thickness burns greater than 20% of BSA in all other age groups, burns to face, hands and genitals, and/or significant chemical burns, electrical burns or inhalational injury.

What is the normal range of carboxyhaemoglobin in the blood?

> Non-smoker   0.3–2%
> Smoker   5–6%.

What are the features of CO poisoning?

Symptoms of CO poisoning vary according to the percentage HbCO present, but no dose–response relationship has been found. Levels, therefore, do not predict outcome.

> 0–10%   None
> 10–20%   Headache, malaise
> 30–40%   Nausea, vomiting, impaired mental ability
> 60–70%   Cardiovascular collapse and death

What is the half-life of HbCO?

> In air: 4–5 hours
> In 100% oxygen: 1 hour
> In hyperbaric oxygen at 3 atmosphere: 30 min.

What are the current criteria for hyperbaric oxygen therapy?

> HbCO >40%
> Neurological symptoms or loss of consciousness
> Arrhythmias or myocardial infarction
> Pregnancy.

50. BRAINSTEM DEATH AND ORGAN DONATION

Brainstem death (BSD) refers to the irreversible absence of normal brainstem functioning. In the UK, BSD equates to human death and this is based on the concept that without brainstem function, higher cerebral activity and conscious perception is deemed impossible.

What are the diagnostic criteria for brainstem death testing?

Before a patient can be certified as BSD, certain preconditions must be met:
> The patient must be in an apnoeic coma and ventilator dependent.
> Irreversible brain damage of known cause must be established.
> Reversible causes of reduced consciousness must be identified and corrected (e.g. hypoxia, hypercapnia, hypothermia, hypotension, acid–base abnormalities, metabolic disturbances (e.g. hyponatraemia), endocrine disease (e.g. hypothyroidism), drugs (e.g. sedative agents and muscle relaxants)).

Only once these preconditions have been met and at least 6 hours have elapsed since the onset of coma can formal BSD testing begin.

Who can perform BSD testing?

The test requires two doctors who have been fully registered with the GMC for at least 5 years, one of whom should be a consultant. Neither should be a member of the organ retrieval team. Each doctor should perform one set of tests, watched by the other. The two sets of tests can be done one after the other and although many choose to wait a few hours in between sets, this is not a legal necessity. Death is legally declared after the completion of the first set of tests.

Which tests are performed?

Several cranial nerves (CN) pathways integrating within the brainstem are tested in order to establish loss of brainstem reflexes to the following:

> **Pupillary light reflex:**
  • Pupils must be fixed, dilated and unresponsive to light.
  • Afferent pathway via optic nerve (CN II) and efferent pathway via parasympathetic fibres carried in the oculomotor nerve (CN III).

> **Corneal reflex:**
>   • No reaction.
>   • Afferent pathway via ophthalmic branch of trigeminal nerve (CN V) and efferent pathway via facial nerve (CN VII).

> **Painful stimulus to the face** (e.g. supra-orbital pressure):
>   • No response should be elicited.
>   • Afferent pathway via trigeminal (CN V) and efferent pathway via facial nerve (CN VII).

> **Vestibulo-ocular reflex** (caloric test):
>   • 30 mL very cold saline is injected rapidly into each external auditory meatus in an attempt to induce nystagmus. If the reflex pathway is intact, the eyes move towards the ipsilateral ear. In the event of BSD there are no eye movements. NB: Examine the auditory canal before performing this test to ensure it is not blocked with wax.
>   • Afferent pathway is via vestibulocochlear nerve (CN VIII) and efferent pathway is via CN III and abducens nerve (CN VI).

> **Gag reflex:**
>   • No gag or cough should be elicited on stimulation of the posterior pharyngeal wall.
>   • Tests glossopharyngeal (CN IX) and vagus nerve (CN X).

> **Apnoea test:** Ventilate the patient with 100% O_2 for 10 min, to ensure normocapnia, then disconnect them from the ventilator. Insufflate O_2, using a tracheal catheter placed down the endotracheal tube, to keep oxygen saturations ≥90%. Watch for respiratory effort during this period. Allow the $PaCO_2$ to increase to 6.65 kP$_a$ before terminating the test. CO_2 rises at approximately 0.5 kP$_a$ per minute during apnoea; levels should be confirmed with a blood gas.

How will you manage the patient following brainstem testing?

If the patient is not brainstem dead, medical care should continue as before.

If the patient is brainstem dead, either:
> Preparations should be made to withdraw life support or
> If the patient is being considered for organ donation, the transplant team will co-ordinate ongoing care until organ harvesting can take place.

At all stages, it is vital that the family be kept informed of events and supported through them.

Organ donation

What are the different types of organ donation?

There are two categories of organ donation:
1 Donation after brainstem death (DBD)
2 Donation after cardiac death (DCD)

Can you describe the principles of each process?

While there are obvious differences in these two processes, they do have common themes:

> The patient must be treated in their best interests at all times. Best interests does not just refer to medical best interests but includes all other emotional and welfare issues. The fact that the patient may be a potential organ donor must not colour decisions about their ongoing medical care.

> Check to see if the patient was on the organ donor register, as this will help inform discussions with the family.

> When considering a patient as a potential organ donor, the family must be consulted early and treated with respect and consideration throughout the process. If they agree to organ donation, they have the right to change their minds at any stage. It is probably best that the opening discussions are lead by the transplant coordinators as they are skilled at navigating the issues in this potentially delicate subject area.

> There is no upper or lower age limit for the donor.

> There are few absolute contraindications to donation, these are:
  • Active invasive cancer within 3 years (excluding non-melanoma skin cancer and brain tumours)
  • Haematological malignancy
  • Untreated systemic infection
  • Variant Creutzfeldt–Jakob disease
  • HIV disease (though not necessarily infection).

Donation after brainstem death (DBD)

Once BSD has been confirmed and consent given by the family, the ongoing care of the decreased donor turns to focus on optimising the condition of the organs while awaiting their retrieval.

Organ damage follows BSD as part of an organic pathophysiological process. Rising intracranial pressure renders the brainstem ischaemic and causes bradycardia and hypertension. As the brainstem infarcts, there is an unregulated surge in autonomic activity and massive catecholamine release, the so-called 'sympathetic storm'.

The hypothalamic–pituitary axis (HA) also fails leading to a decline in hormone levels. These events result in:

> Diabetes insipidus
> Disseminated intravascular coagulation
> Cardiac ischaemia and arrhythmias
> Pulmonary oedema
> Metabolic acidosis
> Hypothermia

Immunological effects are also seen and the immunogenicity of the solid organs increases once BSD occurs in processes that are poorly understood.

To preserve the organs in good condition, it is important to maintain optimal:

> Organ perfusion
> Ventilation
> Hormone replacement with vasopressin, T3, steroids and insulin
> Normal electrolyte status

DBD organ retrieval always seems to take place in the early hours of the morning when everything else on the CEPOD list is finished. There is variation in the approach taken by anaesthetists in these cases. Some give no anaesthetic at all to the donor while others will ventilate with a volatile. The rationale of the latter group is to depress any spinal reflexes that may occur during surgery, and not as a result of concerns about awareness in the donor. These cases can often feel a little unnerving on the first couple of occasions, but the organ retrieval team will usually guide the anaesthetist as to what they need.

Donation after cardiac death

The need for transplantable organs greatly outstrips the supply, and so we have begun to look beyond those who have suffered BSDs. This has lead to the advent of donation after cardiac death, sometimes referred to as non-heart-beating organ donation.

DCD should be considered in all patients where it is decided that further treatment is futile and it is in their best interests to withdraw life-sustaining therapy. By the nature of the process, most of these patients will be on the ICU, but this need not always be the case. The decisions around withdrawal of therapy must be totally separate from any consideration of the patient as an organ donor in the minds of the medical team.

Once life-sustaining therapy has been withdrawn, the donor's organs are subject to 'warm ischaemia'. Warm ischaemia begins when the systolic BP drops below 50 and oxygen saturations fall below 70% and ends when the retrieval team begins to cool the organs that have been removed. This begins the period of 'cold ischaemia', which aims to extend the time of organ preservation.

It is vital that the warm ischaemic time is minimal; a liver must not have a warm ischaemic time of longer than 30 minutes, while the kidneys are more robust and can tolerate 2 hours. In this way, it is possible that a patient may die 'too slowly' following withdrawal of treatment for their organs to be viable for donation.

The organ retrieval team should be gathered and a theatre ready before treatment is withdrawn. The withdrawal process should be managed exactly as normal and no changes should be made because the patient is a potential donor. Death is confirmed by a member of the organ retrieval team when there has been 5 minutes of cardiorespiratory arrest. This must be demonstrated on the ECG or arterial line trace: a finger on the pulse is not sufficient. Surgery does not start until 10 minutes after death to ensure a safety margin. Ten minutes has been chosen because there is no evidence that return of spontaneous circulation has ever happened in any patient who has been in asystole for more than 7 minutes, even with resuscitation attempts. During this time, the family can be with the patient if they wish.

The family should be counselled before about the possibility that if the warm ischaemic time is prolonged, organ retrieval may not be possible; however, tissue and corneas may still be taken.

Part 03

CRITICAL INCIDENTS

51. ANAPHYLAXIS

Anaphylaxis is an acute, Type 1 hypersensitivity reaction caused by antigens binding to IgE immunoglobulin on mast cells and causing them to degranulate. These mast cells release 'anaphylatoxins', mainly histamine, prostaglandins and leukotrienes. It is these mediators that are responsible for the physiological effects of anaphylaxis – vasodilatation, increased capillary permeability and smooth muscle constriction.

In order to undergo an anaphylactic reaction the patient must have been previously sensitised to the antigen (in this context, a drug). However, there are increasing reports of cross-sensitivity between environmental pathogens and anaesthetic agents, especially the non-depolarising muscle relaxants such as rocuronium, meaning that a patient can undergo anaphylaxis following their first exposure to the drug.

What are the signs in an anaesthetised patient?

> Flushing and weals.
> Wheezing, bronchospasm and rising airway pressures, which can make ventilation difficult.
> Oedema of face, lips and oropharynx, which may precipitate airway obstruction.
> Pulmonary oedema may also develop compounding hypoxia.
> Hypotension, which may become profound with complete circulatory collapse.
> Tachycardia.

Differential diagnosis:
Other causes of the same symptoms must be ruled out, for example:
> Haemorrhage
> Asthma
> High regional block
> Myocardial infarction
> MH

The temporal nature of events may aid diagnosis of anaphylaxis.

How would you manage a case of suspected anaphylaxis?

> **Immediate management:**
  • State that this is an anaesthetic emergency and that you need to call for senior anaesthetic assistance.
  • Stop giving the offending drug.
  • Secure the airway and give 100% oxygen.
  • If the patient is paralysed, maintain anaesthesia using inhalational agent (volatiles are not associated with anaphylaxis).
  • Administer adrenaline 50–100 µg IV (0.5–1 mL of 1:10 000 solution).
  • Repeat this dose every minute until there is an improvement in symptoms or deterioration to cardiac arrest, in which case move onto the advanced life support algorithm.
  • Give crystalloid or colloid IV to increase circulating volume.
  • If possible, elevate the patient's legs to improve central blood volume.

> **Early management:**
> • Give antihistamines – chlorpheniramine 10 mg IV.
> • Administer steroids – hydrocortisone 200 mg IV.
> • Administer regular bronchodilators if necessary.
> • Consider inotrope or vasopressor infusion if indicated – adrenaline or noradrenaline.
> • Administer bicarbonate if the patient is severely acidotic.
> • At 1 hour, take blood for serum tryptase levels.
> • Admit to ITU and leave intubated if the airway or ventilation is of concern.
> • Check for a cuff leak prior to extubation.

Put 10 mL of blood into a plain glass tube and send straight to the laboratory where it needs to be stored at −20 °C. An elevated serum tryptase level confirms mast cell degranulation and therefore anaphylaxis.

> **Subsequent management:**
> • It is the responsibility of the anaesthetist involved in the case to refer the patient to an immunologist for further allergy testing.
> • A yellow card (found in the back of the BNF) should also be completed to report the adverse reaction.
> • Document events in the notes, inform the patient of events, send a letter to the GP and complete a critical incident form.

52. ASPIRATION

Aspiration is defined as the inhalation of oropharyngeal or gastric contents into the lower airways. Inhalation can lead to aspiration pneumonitis and/or aspiration pneumonia. The 4th National Audit Project (NAP 4), published in 2011, found that aspiration remained the leading cause of airway-related anaesthetic deaths, with most cases having identifiable risk factors.

Aspiration pneumonitis is an acute, chemically induced inflammation of the lung parenchyma caused by the acid in the gastric contents. The extent of the damage depends on the volume and acidity of the material inhaled. If the damage is severe following this mechanism of lung injury, it is called Mendelson's syndrome, and forms one of the diseases on the ARDS spectrum. Aspiration pneumonitis does not necessarily lead to aspiration pneumonia, and therefore antibiotic prophylaxis has now fallen from favour following simple aspiration.

Aspiration pneumonia occurs when superimposed infection follows aspiration. It is most commonly seen in patients who suffer long-term 'silent' aspiration, e.g. those with neurological problems causing decreased airway protection. However, it may occur following an acute aspiration if the inhaled material is colonised with upper airway flora or in those patients with bowel obstruction whose gastric contents may be colonised with bacteria.

What are the risk factors for aspiration?

Factors that predispose to aspiration may be divided into patient factors and surgical factors.

> **Patient factors:**
> * Reduced level of consciousness – anaesthesia, intoxication, head injury
> * Full stomach – recent meal, pain, trauma, opiates, bowel obstruction, pregnancy, upper GI bleed
> * Reduced barrier pressure – pregnancy, abdominal distension, hiatus hernia, obesity
> * Anatomy – pharyngeal pouch, oesophageal strictures.
> **Surgical factors:**
> * Operation – gastrointestinal surgery
> * Position – lithotomy or head down

How would you manage a case of intra-operative aspiration?

> **Pre-operative:** Management starts with prevention, and this begins with identifying at-risk patients, followed by implementation of risk-reduction strategies:
> * Administration of antacids – e.g. ranitidine or sodium citrate
> * Administration of prokinetic drugs – e.g. metoclopramide
> * Postponing anaesthesia for 6 hours following a meal

> **Peri-operative:**
> - NG tube placement and aspiration of gastric contents prior to surgery
> - Use of rapid sequence induction with cricoid pressure where appropriate
> - Positioning the patient head up where possible.
> **Management of aspiration:**
> - Call for help.
> - Suction the airway.
> - Administer 100% O_2.
> - If possible, place patient in the left lateral position with head down.
> - Intubate if necessary.
> - Suction down the ETT once *in situ* before giving positive-pressure ventilation, if possible. Consider bronchoscopy and bronchial lavage
> - CXR.
> - Transfer to an appropriate bed, e.g. HDU or ITU, for supportive treatment – O_2, bronchodilators and physiotherapy. In severe cases CPAP or IPPV with PEEP may be required post-operatively.
> - Consider antibiotics.
> - Treatment with steroids has not been shown to improve outcome and so is not recommended.
> **Antibiotics:** Antibiotics should be considered if any aspiration pneumonitis does not resolve within 48 hours, if the patient had bowel obstruction or if they have been on regular antacids as the resulting increased pH allows colonisation of the stomach. Each hospital will have its own antibiotic policy regarding aspiration, and microbiology advice should be sought.
> **Starvation protocols:** Patients should be fasted for the following times:
> - Food: 6 hours
> - Clear fluid: 2 hours
> - Breast milk: 4 hours
> - Bottle formula: 6 hours
> - Milk: 6 hours
> - Chewing gum: 2 hours

Clear fluid: if you are able to read the typed page through the fluid, it counts as clear. More sugar-laden fluids such as cola count as food.

53. AWARENESS

Awareness is currently one of the most common pre-operative anxieties expressed by patients for whom awareness under general anaesthesia is a terrifying experience that can result in debilitating psychological sequelae and even post-traumatic stress disorder. For the anaesthetist, it can also lead to serious consequences with medico-legal claims for awareness constituting 2% of all claims made against American anaesthetists. The 5th National Audit project (NAP 5), published in 2012, is the largest study in the world that looked at the incidence and mechanism of accidental awareness under general anesthesia (AAGA). Figures quoted here are from the NAP 5 data.

What do you understand by the term awareness?

Awareness under general anaesthesia is the ability to perceive, feel or be consciously aware of one's surroundings; this may or may not be accompanied by the experience of pain. There are two types of awareness:

> Explicit memory (or recall). This is the intentional recollection of events with conscious perception.
> Implicit memory (or recall). This is the non-intentional recollection of events with subconscious perception (i.e. these patients may remember events under hypnosis).

What is the incidence of awareness?

NAP 5 data gave an estimated overall incidence of AAGA of 1:19 000 anaesthetics. The incidence varied considerably depending on the setting: 1:670 for obstetric rapid sequence inductions, 1:8000 when a neuromuscular blockade was used (vs. 1:136 000 without it) and 1:8600 in cardiothoracic anaesthesia.

What are the risk factors associated with awareness?

> **Phase of anaesthesia:**
  • Induction and emergence account for two-thirds of all reported AAGA cases.
  • Interrupting delivery of anaesthesia to transfer patients from the anaesthetic room into theatre is also a time of risk.
> **Anaesthetic drugs and techniques:**
  • Neuromuscular blocking drugs-incidence increases from 1:136 000 to 1:8000. On emergence, failure to use a nerve stimulator to ensure adequate return of muscle power before turning off anaesthetic agents is a major contributory factor to AAGA.
  • Total intravenous anaesthesia – no real-time plasma concentration of intravenous agent can be made and therefore pharmacokinetic models are relied upon to 'predict' plasma and effect site concentrations.
  • Thiopental is associated with an increased incidence.
  • Rapid sequence induction.

- Inadequate administration of volatile agent – MAC is the minimum alveolar concentration, at one atmosphere ambient pressure, required to prevent movement in 50% of subjects in response to a surgical stimulus. The definition does not encompass the concept of awareness, only movement. There is now substantial evidence to suggest a correlation between MAC and recall, with explicit recall being extremely unlikely at MAC > 1. However, MAC is influenced by a variety of factors and published data for MAC is typically quoted for healthy, unmedicated subjects. All of these factors must be taken into consideration when interpreting MAC values.
- Drug error – this accounted for 10% of the reports of AAGA to NAP5.

> **Patient factors**
  - Female
  - Younger adults (but not children)
  - Obesity
  - Previous AAGA
  - Patients who are unexpectedly difficult to intubate
  - Patients with increased resistance to anaesthetic agents including those that are febrile, hyperthyroid, alcoholic and or use recreational drugs
  - Moribund patients for emergency procedures

> **Subspecialities:**
  - Obstetrics (includes most of the risk factors: emergency, rapid sequence induction, thiopental, neuromuscular blockade, high incidence of obesity and difficult intubations)
  - Cardiothoracics (patients on cardiopulmonary bypass or those undergoing bronchoscopies)

> **Equipment:**
  - Faulty or malfunctioning equipment
  - Equipment not used or programmed correctly by the anaesthetist

> **Monitoring:**
  - Failure to monitor concentration of inspired and expired volatile agents and MAC
  - Failure to monitor peripheral cannula and infusion line with TIVA
  - Failure to use specific depth of anaesthesia monitoring (e.g. entropy, BIS etc.)
  - Failure to look for clinical signs of awareness (heart rate, blood pressure, tachypnoea, sweating and lacrimation)
  - Absence of clinical signs of awareness due to drugs (e.g. β-blockers will mask a tachycardia and hypertension, anti-muscarinic agents will mask sweating and tear production, opioids will mask pupillary dilation and neuromuscular blockers will mask movement and tachypnoea)

What would you do if a patient complains they were aware under general anaesthesia?

This is a serious situation with potentially devastating consequences to both the patient and anaesthetist involved. NAP 5 suggested that 41% of patients reporting AAGA experienced moderate or severe long-term sequelae. Early reassurance and support often led to good outcomes. Seek advice from a consultant.

> Visit the patient as soon as possible with a witness (preferably a consultant).
> Take a full history and elicit exactly what the patient sensed and whether they were in pain.

> Document all conversations.
> Review the medical notes and anaesthetic records and try to ascertain the cause.
> Be sympathetic and if true awareness is suspected, apologise.
> Give a full explanation to the patient.
> Offer a follow-up appointment and psychological support. Reassure patient that this is very unlikely to happen again.
> Inform patient's GP, the hospital administrators and your medical defence organisation.
> Complete a critical incident form.
> Debrief with your consultant to try to determine what, if anything, could have been done differently.

54. BLOOD TRANSFUSION ERROR

What steps should be taken to minimise the risk of administering incorrect blood products to a patient?

The Blood Transfusion Task Force has issued guidelines on the process of red cell transfusion. A summary of these recommendations is as follows:

Once the decision to transfuse has been made, the following procedures should be followed to minimise the incorrect administration of red cells to the patient:

> All staff involved in blood transfusions must have undergone mandatory training in blood transfusion safety.
> Decisions concerning the need to transfuse the patient should be documented in the medical notes.
> Identity of the patient must be confirmed (four standard identifiers required: first name, surname, date of birth and hospital/NHS number).
> Samples must not be accepted by the laboratory without the correct four standard identifiers.
> Blood compatibility label must be checked to ensure that the blood is correct for the patient.
> Expiry date should be checked.
> Bag should be inspected to ensure integrity of the plastic casing.
> Removed patient identification bands must be replaced or reattached.
> Blood left out of a blood fridge for longer than 30 minutes should be transfused within 4 hours or discarded.
> Details of the unit of blood transfused should be recorded on the anaesthetic chart or in the contemporaneous clinical notes.
> Tear-off sticky labels may facilitate this data recording.
> Volume of blood transfused should be recorded once administered.
> 100% traceability of all allogeneic blood transfused is a legal requirement following the European Blood Directive.
> Good communication between the medical staff and the laboratory is essential.

Failure to adhere to the above recommendations increases the chances of a transfusion error occurring. Blood transfusion errors are also evaluated by the Serious Hazards Of Transfusion (SHOT). SHOT is based at the Manchester Blood Transfusion Centre and is affiliated to the Royal College of Pathologists. Among its many roles, it aims to build an evidence base of transfusion hazards and encourage UK hospitals to participate in haemovigilance. SHOT is now entering its second decade of reporting as one of the longest established haemovigilance systems in the world. Mortality from blood transfusion is low, but there is avoidable major morbidity. In 2007 there were 12 severe (anaphylactic) cases of ABO-incompatible red cell transfusion, 9 arising from clinical error and 3 from laboratory error. SABRE (Serious Adverse Blood Reaction and Events) is an online system submission of notification and subsequent confirmation of blood-related adverse events and reactions.

What is an acute haemolytic transfusion reaction?

If blood is mistakenly administered to the wrong patient, the chances of ABO incompatibility are approximately one in three. The reaction is usually most severe if Group A cells are transfused to a Group O patient. Incompatible transfused cells react with the patient's own anti-A or anti-B antibodies or other alloantibodies (e.g. Kell/Duffy) to red cell antigens. This reaction can lead to activation of complement and cause disseminated intravascular coagulation (DIC).

Infusion of ABO incompatible blood still almost always arises from errors in labelling the sample tube or the cross-match request form or from inadequate checks when blood is administered.

What are the symptoms and signs of a haemolytic transfusion reaction?

In a conscious patient even a few millilitres of ABO-incompatible blood may cause symptoms (agitation, pain at infusion site, flushing, abdominal, flank or substernal pain and breathlessness) within 1–2 minutes.

Signs may include pyrexia, hypotension, bleeding, haemoglobinaemia and haemoglobinuria.

In an unconscious or anaesthetised patient hypotension and uncontrollable bleeding secondary to DIC may be the only signs of an incompatible transfusion.

How would you manage an acute haemolytic transfusion reaction?

ABO incompatibility/acute haemolytic transfusion reaction is a medical emergency that requires prompt recognition and management.

If an acute haemolytic transfusion reaction is suspected, the transfusion must be stopped and urgent steps be taken to confirm or exclude this possibility. The differential diagnosis must include infusion of bacterially contaminated blood.

State that this is an anaesthetic emergency and that you would call for senior anaesthetic assistance.

> Adopt an ABC approach.
> Stop the blood transfusion and administer colloid.
> Support respiration and circulation as necessary with supplemental oxygen, bronchodilators, volume resuscitation and consider adrenaline, vasopressors and chlorpheniramine.
> Check that the compatibility label of the blood unit corresponds with the patient's ID bands, blood forms and case-notes.
> If a mistake is discovered, inform blood bank urgently since the unit of blood intended for your patient could be given out to transfuse another patient.
> Inform the consultant haematologist.
> If clinical evidence of DIC develops, transfuse platelets, fresh frozen plasma and cryoprecipitate guided by clinical state and coagulation study results.
> If the patient requires red cell transfusion, repeat cross-match.
> If bacterial contamination is suspected, administer broad-spectrum IV antibiotics.
> Take 35 mL blood for:
>   • Haematology – 5 mL EDTA tube – FBC, platelet count, direct antiglobulin test (DAT) and plasma haemoglobin
>   • 5 mL in a dry tube for repeat cross-matching
>   • 10 mL in a citrated tube – for coagulation screen (PT, APTT, fibrinogen)
>   • Clinical chemistry – 5 mL for urea and electrolytes
> Take blood cultures.
> Return blood packs and giving set to blood bank for bacteriology.
> Urine dip – haemoglobinuria.

> ABG – metabolic acidosis and hyperkalaemia.
> Monitor ECG – for changes suggestive of hyperkalaemia (from haemolysis).
> Maintain urine output to minimise risk of acute kidney injury.
> Liaise with critical care, if indicated.
> Complete hospital critical incident reporting forms.
> Report incident to SABRE.

Can haemolytic reactions occur due to red cell antibodies other than ABO?

Haemolytic reactions can be caused by other red cell antibodies in the recipient's blood, including anti Rh D, Rh E, Rh C and K (Kell).

Reactions due to anti D are rare since patients generally receive Rh D–compatible red cells. Reactions due to these antibodies are usually less severe than those caused by ABO incompatibility since they do not activate complement. Destruction of transfused red cells occurs mainly in the liver and spleen. The patient may experience fever, nausea and shivering.

However, the Kidd and Duffy antigens do activate complement and can cause severe intravascular haemolysis leading to cardiac and renal failure. Kidd antibodies are often difficult to find in pre-transfusion samples.

A falling haemoglobin or a rise in haemoglobin that is less than expected after transfusion together with a rise in bilirubin and a positive direct antiglobulin test indicates that red cells are being destroyed.

55. BRADYCARDIA

As soon as you are presented with a critical incident, you must be thinking of the most probable causes and how you will identify and manage them. You must be systematic in your thought process so that you do not miss anything out, as this could potentially be fatal to your patient (and thus to your performance). Your answers must be confident and to the point, because in a real-life situation time is of the essence.

What is the definition of bradycardia?

In an adult a bradycardia is defined as an HR <60 bpm, but in reality you should take into consideration any rate that is inappropriately slow for that individual and haemodynamic state.

What are the causes of intra-operative bradycardia?

> **Hypoxia:** This is the most important cause.
> **Vagal stimulation:** This can be caused during eye surgery, dilation of the anus and cervix, mesenteric retraction, laparoscopy and airway manipulation.
> **Drugs:**
> • Inhalational agents (enflurane and halothane > isoflurane)
> • Opioids (fentanyl, remifentanil and morphine)
> • Anticholinesterases (neostigmine)
> • Muscle relaxants (vecuronium, tubocurarine and second dose of suxamethonium)
> • Vasopressors (metaraminol and phenylephrine can cause a reflex bradycardia)
> • β-Blockers that patient may be on pre-operatively
> **Neuroaxial blocks:** High spinal blockade to T1–T4 will compromise the cardiac sympathetic accelerator fibres.
> **Metabolic:** Hypothyroidism and hyperkalaemia.
> **Disease:** Ischaemic heart disease and raised intracranial pressure.
> **Normal:** Athletes.

How would you manage an anaesthetised patient who developed bradycardia intra-operatively?

Remember that you need to assess and resuscitate the patient simultaneously, using an ABC approach and systematically work your way from the patient back towards the anaesthetic machine so as not to miss anything. The haemodynamic consequences of the bradycardia will determine the urgency of the situation.

> **Immediate management:**
> • State that this is an anaesthetic emergency and that you would call for senior anaesthetic assistance.
> • Ask the surgeon to stop as this will eliminate any surgical vagal stimulation.
> • Administer 100% oxygen and hand-ventilate the patient. This allows you to assess lung compliance and adequacy of ventilation.

- Reduce or even stop the volatile agent. Check the MAC and end-tidal concentration of the volatile agent.
- Administer atropine 0.6 mg (10 µg/kg) and flush. Repeat if necessary up to a maximum of 3 mg.
- Check BP and if hypotensive give fluid bolus (10 mL/kg of either crystalloid or colloid). Repeat if necessary. Bolus vasopressors agents, e.g. ephedrine, as required.
- If there is no satisfactory response, reassess the situation starting at ABC and treat the probable cause as appropriate.

> **Management options in persistent bradycardia:**
  - Ask for the crash trolley.
  - Administer adrenaline 2–10 µg/min of 1:10 000 preparation.
  - Commence transcutaneous pacing (this can be done using defibrillator chest pads with the defibrillator machine set to pacing mode at a rate of 50–60 bpm). Expert help will later be needed to arrange transvenous pacing.
  - If HR <30 with significant haemodynamic compromise, commence CPR and follow ALS algorithm for asystole.
  - Terminate surgery as soon as safely possible.
  - Arrange transfer to ICU for further investigation, advanced monitoring and management.
  - Document sequence of events in medical notes.
  - Complete a critical incident form.

56. CYANOSIS

Cyanosis describes the blue discolouration of the skin and mucous membranes due to the presence of increased quantities of deoxygenated haemoglobin. The name is derived from the Greek word 'cyan' for blue.

Cyanosis becomes clinically evident when arterial oxygen saturations fall below approximately 85–90%; this correlates with a deoxyhaemoglobin level of at least 5 g/dL.

This answer should be read in conjunction with critical incidents on hypoxia and difficult to ventilate.

How can you classify cyanosis?

Cyanosis can be classified as central or peripheral.

> **Central cyanosis:**
> • Most visible in the tongue and lips
> • Commonest causes are cardio-respiratory problems, which may be acute (e.g. obstructed airway) or chronic (e.g. some types of congenital heart disease).
> **Peripheral cyanosis:**
> • Visible in the fingers and nail beds
> • Caused by reduced peripheral perfusion
> • May be seen in combination with central cyanosis.

What are the causes of congenital cyanotic heart disease?

Cyanosis occurs in patients with congenital heart lesions that result in a right to left shunt of blood:

> Tetralogy of Fallot
> Pulmonary stenosis or atresia with septal defect
> Truncus arteriosus
> Total anomalous pulmonary venous drainage
> Transposition of the great arteries.

What are the common causes of peripheral cyanosis?

> All of the causes of central cyanosis
> Cold-induced peripheral vasoconstriction
> Raynaud's phenomenon
> Low cardiac output states (e.g. cardiac failure).

In terms of relevance to anaesthesia, the most important cause of cyanosis is hypoxia, due to airway or ventilatory compromise until proven otherwise.

57. DIFFICULT TO VENTILATE (HIGH AIRWAY PRESSURES)

This is a relatively common critical incident exam question. The ability to manage this event effectively in the clinical setting requires a clear systematic approach to the problem.

What factors may cause you to experience difficulty ventilating an anaesthetised patient intra-operatively?

This can be classified into patient factors and non-patient factors.

Patient factors:
> Reduced chest wall compliance:
  - Chest wall rigidity, malignant hyperthermia or opioids
  - Prone position
  - Obesity
  - Kyphoscoliosis
  - Raised abdominal pressures, e.g. pneumoperitoneum
  - Inadequate paralysis or patient 'fighting' ventilator.
> Reduced lung compliance:
  - Pneumothorax
  - Bronchospasm
  - Lobar collapse or atelectasis
  - Pulmonary oedema
  - Pulmonary fibrosis
  - Aspiration
  - ARDS

Non-patient factors:
> Anaesthetic circuit:
  - Blockage, compression, kinking of tubing
  - Incorrect connection of circuit, scavenging, reservoir bag, filter, humidifier, APL valve or PEEP valve.
> Ventilator:
  - Excessive tidal volumes.
> Endotracheal tube:
  - Kinked
  - Misplaced, e.g. oesophageal or endobronchial
  - Obstructed, e.g. sputum, blood or foreign body

Treat the identified cause, clearly document the sequence of events on the anaesthetic chart and complete a critical incident form.

How would you identify such a case?

Presentation:
> Difficult to ventilate
> Decreased compliance in reservoir bag, poor chest expansion, low minute volume
> High airway pressure and alarm limits reached
> Abnormal CO_2 trace
> Hypoxia
> Circulatory collapse

Describe your management.

State that this is an anaesthetic emergency, and that you would call for senior anaesthetic assistance.

> ABC approach: assess and resuscitate simultaneously.
> Check the basic parameters: heart rate, ECG, blood pressure, oxygen saturation, $ETCO_2$ trace.
> Hand-ventilate with 100% oxygen.
> Ask the surgeon to stop operating until it is safe to continue.
> Exclude obvious causes: start at the patient (check tube position and auscultate chest) and sequentially examine from the airway back to the anaesthetic machine. Treat the cause as you discover it. Consider switching to an alternative circuit, e.g. Ambu bag.

Consider the context:
> Patient position: prone, Trendelenburg
> Pre-existing disease: asthma, obesity, ARDS
> Timing of event: e.g. following central venous line insertion
> Risk factors: allergy, bronchospasm
> Surgery: e.g. laparoscopy with pneumoperitoneum.

58. FAILED INTUBATION

Failed intubations occur in approximately 1:2000 elective intubations, 1:300 obstetric rapid sequence intubations and 1:50–100 intubations in the ICU or emergency department. Patients do not die from lack of intubation but from lack of ventilation and oxygenation, and all too often the anaesthetist becomes fixated on trying to intubate at the expense of resuscitating the hypoxic patient. The Difficult Airway Society (DAS) has published guidelines on how to manage 'the failed intubation' scenario. You will be expected to know these as examiners are likely to take a very harsh view of faltering knowledge in this crucial area.

What is a difficult intubation?

A difficult intubation is defined as one in which an anaesthetist with at least 2 years' training, using a traditional laryngoscope blade, achieves only a poor view at direct laryngoscopy (grade 3 or 4) *or* requires more than three attempts at direct laryngoscopy *or* more than 10 minutes to intubate *or* additional equipment in order to secure the airway. Difficult intubations are thought to occur in about 1 in 65 cases.

What patient factors contribute to a difficult intubation?

> **Congenital**, e.g. Down's, Pierre Robin, Treacher Collins and Marfan's syndromes
> **Anatomical**, e.g. morbid obesity, pregnancy, large breasts, thick, short and immobile necks, protruding teeth, beards and receding jaws
> **Disease**, e.g. acromegaly, scleroderma, rheumatoid arthritis, airway malignancy and cervical spine fractures
> **Acquired**, e.g. swelling, infection, trauma and scars

How can you predict if a patient is likely to be difficult to intubate?

Unfortunately, there is no single test that can predict all difficult intubations and despite pre-operative airway evaluation, 20% of all difficult intubations are not predicted. An anaesthetic airway assessment should encompass the following:

Review the medical records and previous anaesthetic charts:
> Cormack and Lehane grade: establish previous grade of intubation (grade 3 or 4 is considered difficult) and any airway complications.

History:
> **Presenting pathology:** e.g. airway malignancies are likely to be associated with a difficult airway.
> **Medical diseases:** e.g. rheumatoid arthritis can affect the temporomandibular joints, neck and arytenoids.
> **Surgery to the neck and airway:** this can distort airway anatomy.
> **Radiotherapy to the head and neck:** this can distort airway anatomy and cause tissues surrounding the airway to become rigid, making head extension, jaw thrust and direct laryngoscopy very difficult.
> **Anaesthesia:** ask the patient whether they had any problems, such as dental damage during previous anaesthetics.

Examination:
> **General:**
  * BMI
  * Beard (often covers a small, receding chin)
  * Large breasts (makes inserting the laryngoscope difficult; consider using a short-handle laryngoscope)
> **Head and neck:**
  * Scars
  * Swellings (e.g. goitre)
  * Burns or radiotherapy
  * Range of neck movement
> **Inter-incisor gap:**
  * Normal should be 5 cm or three-finger breaths (using patient's own fingers).
> **Mallampati score:**
  * Performed with patient sitting up, head in neutral position, mouth wide open and tongue protruding with no phonation.
  * Classes I–III were first described by Mallampati in 1983 and class IV was later added by Samsoon and Young in 1987. There is now also a class 0, applicable when you can visualise the epiglottis!
> **Teeth:** Protruding teeth make direct laryngoscopy difficult while the edentulous patient makes face mask ventilation difficult.
> **Tongue:** Large tongues, as seen in patients with Down's syndrome, make inserting the laryngoscope difficult and can obscure the view.
> **Jaw slide:**
  * This gives an indication of the degree of mandibular subluxation that can occur during maximal forward protrusion of the mandible.
  * It is classified as A – lower incisors lie beyond the upper incisors, B – lower incisors meet upper incisors and C – lower incisors remain behind upper incisors.
> **Thyromental distance:** This represents the gap available to displace the tongue and should be ≥6.5 cm.

Radiological investigations:
> CT or MRI of upper airway and neck
> X-ray of mandible and cervical spine

Radiological features that may aid prediction of a difficult intubation include:

> Reduced distance between the occiput and spine of C1
> Reduced distance between spine of C1 and C2
> Ratio of mandibular length to posterior mandibular depth >3.6.

Other investigations:
> **Flexible nasal endoscopy:** Typically performed by ENT surgeons. Good views of the base of the tongue and vocal cords are obtained.
> **Flow–volume loops:** Can help to differentiate between intrinsic and extrinsic causes of stridor.

What is the Wilson risk sum score?

Table 58.1   Wilson risk sum score

Risk factor	Variable	Score
Weight	<90 kg	0
	90–110 kg	1
	>110 kg	2
Head and neck movement	>90°	0
	90°	1
	<90°	2
Jaw movement	Inter-incisor gap ≥5 cm and subluxation = A	0
	Inter-incisor gap <5 cm and subluxation = B	1
	Inter-incisor gap <5 cm and subluxation = C	2
Receding mandible	Normal	0
	Moderate	1
	Severe	2
Protruding teeth	Normal	0
	Moderate	1
	Severe	2

This is a scoring system designed to predict a difficult intubation. It comprises five risk factors each scoring between 0 and 2 points with a maximum total of 10 points:

A score of more than 2 predicts approximately 75% of difficult intubations.

What are the management options of a failed intubation?

In any failed intubation scenario, there are four questions that must be addressed in order to determine the safest management option for the patient:

> **Can the patient be ventilated?**
  - If the patient can be ventilated, this allows time for help to be summoned and intubating aids to be brought.
  - If the patient cannot be ventilated, the 'can't intubate, can't ventilate' algorithm from the DAS should be followed.
> **Is this an RSI or non-RSI technique?**
  - Time constraints and the risk of aspiration may complicate a failed RSI intubation.
> **Is surgery elective or emergency?**
  - If surgery is elective and no immediate assistance is at hand and no advanced airway equipment set up, then the patient should be woken up and alternative options including awake fibre-optic intubation, regional anaesthetic techniques or local anaesthetic techniques should be considered. Alternatively, surgery should be postponed.
  - If immediate surgery is essential because without it the patient would incur serious morbidity or even death, provided the patient can be adequately ventilated, the safest option of maintaining the patient's airway (e.g. LMA ProSeal™) needs to be decided.
  - Remember that the examiners are asking for what *you* would do in this situation. Do not jump the gun and offer them a technique with which you are unfamiliar; tell them which technique would be safest in your hands.
> **Is the patient pregnant?**
  - The mother's survival is paramount.
  - Two situations in which surgery may be required despite failure of intubation are maternal cardiac arrest (CPR is not effective without delivery of the baby) and imminent risk of life to the mother if surgery does not proceed (e.g. massive peri-partum haemorrhage).

Post-operatively:

> The patient should be reviewed.
> The exact nature of the difficult airway must be clearly documented in the anaesthetic notes with particular mention of ease of bag valve mask ventilation.
> The patient must be informed of this and encouraged to alert all future anaesthetists.
> A 'difficult airway alert' form should be completed and given to the patient and a copy sent to the GP (the DAS website has a letter template).

DAS has published guidelines on the management of various 'failed intubation' scenarios. You must be well versed with these algorithms, as any evidence of faltering knowledge is likely to lead to a failure. These guidelines are reproduced with the permission of DAS at the end of this question.

Do you know of any national audits relating to the difficult airway?

The fourth National Audit Project (NAP 4), conducted by the Royal College of Anaesthetists and DAS, was published in 2011 and is the world's largest prospective audit that looked into the incidence of major airway complications within the UK (death, brain damage, surgical or needle cricothyroidotomy and unanticipated ICU admissions related to an airway complication) Data were collected for 1 year between 2008 and 2009. There were two phases to the audit:

> Snapshot phase: Performed over a 2-week period, data on the total numbers and types of anaesthetically related airway interventions were collected. These data were then extrapolated to give the number of airway interventions that were performed within the UK per annum.
> Data collection phase: Performed over a 1-year period, the total number of major airway complications was collected, enabling the incidence of these complications to be calculated (data collected also for ICU and emergency departments).

Major findings of NAP4:

> 2.9 million general anaesthetics were performed in UK NHS hospitals over the 1-year period. The airway management for these cases were as follows:
>   • 56% had a supraglottic airway device (e.g. LMA)
>   • 38% had a tracheal tube
>   • 5% were managed with a face mask
> Poor airway assessment (either incomplete or with omissions) along with a failure to alter the management plan in response to the findings of these assessments contributed to poor airway outcomes.
> Poor airway planning strategies contributed to poor airway outcomes. Anaesthetists must have a logical sequence of plans to manage various airway complications.
> Awake fibre-optic intubations were not always used when indicated.
> Problems arose when difficult intubations were managed by multiple repeat attempts at intubation with no change of approach.
> At least one in four major airway events reported came from ICU or the emergency department.
> Failure to use capnography in ventilated patients was a likely contributing factor in 70% of all ICU-related airway deaths.
> Displaced tracheostomies, and to a lesser extent tracheal tubes, were a major cause of morbidity on ICU.
> Most events in the emergency department were complications of rapid sequence induction.

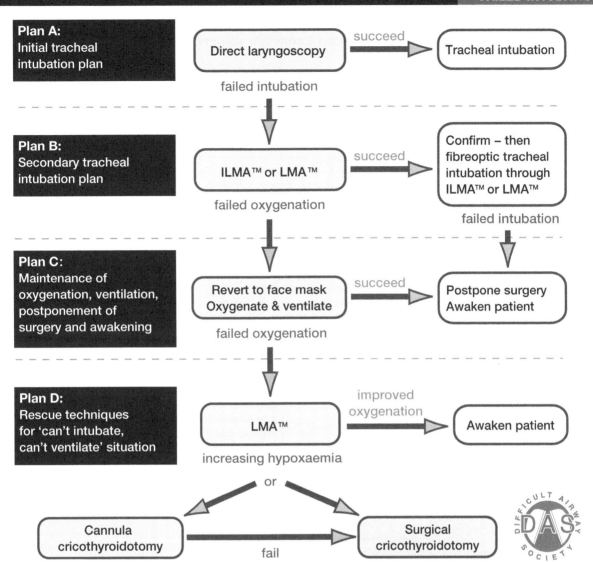

Fig. 58.1   DAS flow chart 1 – Generic sequence of steps that should be taken in a 'failed intubation' scenario

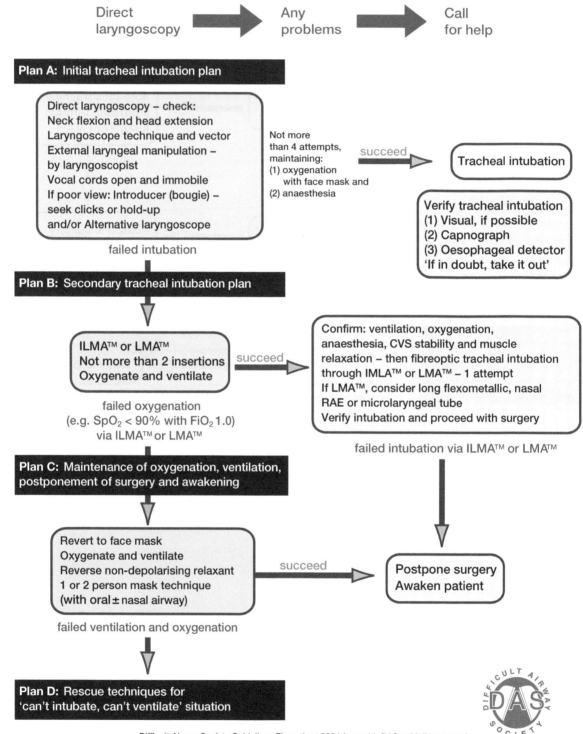

Fig. 58.2   DAS flow chart 2 – Unanticipated difficult intubation during routine induction

Unanticipated difficult tracheal intubation – during rapid sequence
induction of anaestheia in non-obstetric adult patient

Direct laryngoscopy → Any problems → Call for help

Plan A: Initial tracheal intubation plan

Pre-oxygenate
Cricoid force: 10N awake → 30N anaesthetised
Direct laryngoscopy – check:
   Neck flexion and head extension
   Laryngoscopy technique and vector
   External laryngeal manipulation –
   by laryngoscopist
   Vocal cords open and immobile
If poor view:
   Reduce cricoid force
   Introducer (bougie) – seek clicks or hold-up
   and/or Alternative laryngoscope

— succeed → Tracheal intubation

Not more than 3 attempts, maintaining:
(1) oxygenation with face mask
(2) cricoid pressure and
(3) anaesthesia

Verify tracheal intubation
(1) Visual, if possible
(2) Capnograph
(3) Oesophageal detector
'If in doubt, take it out'

failed intubation

Plan C: Maintenance of oxygenation, ventilation, postponement of surgery and awakening

Maintain 30N cricoid force

Plan B not appropriate for this scenario

Use face mask, oxygenate and ventilate
1 or 2 person mask technique
(with oral ± nasal airway)
Consider reducing cricoid force if
ventilation difficult

— succeed →

failed oxygenation
(e.g. SpO$_2$ < 90% with FiO$_2$ 1.0) via face mask

LMA™
Reduce cricoid force during insertion
Oxygenate and ventilate

— succeed →

Postpone surgery
and awaken patient if possible
or continue anaesthesia with
LMA™ or ProSeal LMA™ –
if condition immediately
life-threatening

failed ventilation and oxygenation

Plan D: Rescue techniques for
'can't intubate, can't ventilate' situation

Difficult Airway Society Guidelines Flow-chart 2004 (use with DAS guidelines paper)

Fig. 58.3 DAS flow chart 3 – Unanticipated difficult intubation during rapid sequence induction

Failed intubation, increasing hypoxaemia and difficult ventilation in the paralysed anaesthetised patient: Rescue techniques for the 'can't intubate, can't ventilate' situation

failed intubation and difficult ventilation (other than laryngospasm)

Face mask
Oxygenate and Ventilate patient
Maximum head extension
Maximum jaw thrust
Assistance with mask seal
Oral ± 6 mm nasal airway
Reduce cricoid force – if necessary

failed oxygenation with face mask (e.g. $SpO_2 < 90\%$ with FiO_2 1.0)

call for help

LMA™ Oxygenate and ventilate patient
Maximum 2 attempts at insertion
Reduce any cricoid force during insertion

succeed →

Oxygenation satisfactory and stable: Maintain oxygenation and awaken patient

'can't intubate, can't ventilate' situation with increasing hypoxaemia

Plan D: Rescue techniques for 'can't intubate, can't ventilate' situation

or

Cannula cricothyroidotomy

Equipment: Kink-resistant cannula, e.g. Patil (Cook) or Ravussin (VBM)
High-pressure ventilation system, e.g. Manujet III (VBM)
Technique:
1. Insert cannula through cricothyroid membrane
2. Maintain position of cannula – assistant's hand
3. Confirm tracheal position by air aspiration – 20 ml syringe
4. Attach ventilation system to cannula
5. Commence cautious ventilation
6. Confirm ventilation of lungs, and exhalation through upper airway
7. If ventilation fails, or surgical emphysema or any other complication develops – convert immediately to surgical cricothyroidotomy

fail →

Surgical cricothyroidotomy

Equipment: Scalpel – short and rounded (no. 20 or Minitrach scalpel)
Small (e.g. 6 or 7 mm) cuffed tracheal or tracheostomy tube
4-step Technique:
1. Identify cricothyroid membrane
2. Stab incision through skin and membrane Enlarge incision with blunt dissection (e.g. scalpel handle, forceps or dilator)
3. Caudal traction on cricoid cartilage with tracheal hook
4. Insert tube and inflate cuff
Ventilate with low-pressure source
Verify tube position and pulmonary ventilation

Notes:
1. These techniques can have serious complications – use only in life-threatening situations
2. Convert to definitive airway as soon as possible
3. Postoperative management – see other difficult airway guidelines and flow-charts
4. 4mm cannula with low-pressure ventilation may be successful in patient breathing spontaneously

Difficult Airway Society guidelines Flow-chart 2004 (use with DAS guidelines paper)

Fig. 58.4 DAS flow chart 4 – Rescue techniques for the 'can't intubate, can't ventilate' scenario

59. FAILURE TO BREATHE

Failure to breathe adequately following general anaesthesia requires a systematic approach to its management; the cause must be elucidated and in the interim patient's airway, oxygenation and ventilation maintained.

To establish the cause, approach the problem systematically, remembering all of the requirements for breathing, starting with the central nervous system and ending at the respiratory muscles.

What are the causes of failure to breath post-operatively?

> **Upper airway obstruction:**
  - Foreign body
  - Secretions
  - Oedema
  - Laryngospasm
  - Soft tissue collapse, e.g. obtunded patient or obstructive sleep apnoea
  - Vocal cord palsy
> **Decreased ventilatory drive:**
  - Opiate-induced respiratory depression
  - Presence of inhalational agents
  - Extremes of arterial CO_2 tension
  - Loss of hypoxic drive in COPD patients
  - Acute intracranial catastrophe
> **Inadequate respiratory muscle function:**
  - Incomplete reversal of neuromuscular blocking agents
  - Plasma cholinesterase deficiency
  - High spinal anaesthesia
  - Spinal cord lesion
  - Neuromuscular disease, e.g. myasthenia gravis
  - Restriction due to pain
  - Upper airway obstruction, e.g. foreign body, secretions, oedema, laryngospasm or vocal cord palsy

Some of the causes of failure to breathe are examined further below:

> **Inadequate reversal after non-depolarising neuromuscular blockers has been administered:**
  - Signs may include uncoordinated 'see-saw' breathing movements or inability to sustain a head lift for >5 seconds. Confirm the diagnosis by checking the patient's train-of-four with a nerve stimulator looking for fade, which would indicate a residual block. Also confirm that the correct dose of reversal has been administered.
  - Drugs administered such as magnesium sulphate can increase the duration of neuromuscular blockade.
  - Ensure that the patient is not aware during the period of inadequate reversal.

> **Deranged physiology:** Acidosis and hypothermia may also result in failure of adequate ventilation. Correct these where possible, and if it is not possible acutely, the patient may require a period of post-operative ventilation during which deranged physiology can be corrected.

> **Poor general condition:** Malnourished patients and those with pre-existing conditions causing weakness may not have the muscle strength to sustain adequate ventilation post-operatively and again they may require a period of extended ventilation to allow recovery.

It is important to convey to the examiners a clear thought process and a structure approach to this clinical problem.

60. HIGH SPINAL BLOCK

Spinal anaesthesia is commonly administered to provide dense peri-operative analgesia for surgical procedures involving the abdomen or lower limbs. The spread of intrathecal local anaesthetic above T4 constitutes high spinal anaesthesia.

Total spinal may be defined as intrathecal local anaesthetic-induced depression of the cervical spinal cord and/or brainstem. It may occur secondary to administration of an excessive dose of local anaesthetic or excessive spread of a correct dose.

What factors determine the intrathecal spread of local anaesthetic?

> **Local anaesthetic:** dosage, volume and baricity
> **Patient position**
> **Patient characteristics**, e.g. height, intra-abdominal pressure
> **Injection technique**, e.g. speed of injection, barbotage (i.e. repeated injection and aspiration of the fluid)

What are the clinical features of high spinal blockade?

Clinical features are determined by the height of the block:

> **Cardiovascular:**
> • Hypotension due to vasodilatation
> • Bradycardia may occur due to inhibition of cardio-accelerator fibres (T1–T4).
> **Respiratory:**
> • Intercostal muscle paralysis leading to reduced tidal volumes
> • Block above C3 will involve the diaphragm and may cause respiratory embarrassment
> • Total spinal will involve the brainstem and result in apnoea
> **Neurological:**
> • Total spinal anaesthesia will result in loss of consciousness.
> **Sensory loss:**
> • Paraesthesia in the upper limbs may progress into the face.
> **Motor loss:**
> • Motor loss in the upper limbs indicates high spinal blockade.

A rapidly ascending block may present as cardio-respiratory arrest.

How would you manage a high spinal anaesthetic block?

State that this is an anaesthetic emergency and that you would call for senior anaesthetic assistance.

• Adopt an ABC approach. Management is supportive.
• Administer 100% O_2.
• Monitor adequacy of breathing – consider intubation and ventilation.
• Support the circulation – administration of fluid plus vasopressors, e.g. phenylephrine.
• Treat bradycardia, e.g. atropine/ephedrine.
• Support ventilation and circulation until block has regressed.
• Document the event in the medical notes and complete a critical incident report.
• Inform the patient of the event.

61. HYPERTENSION

Your answer needs to be tailored to the likely cause of the hypertension, and the examiners will lead you in their questioning. Definition of what constitutes 'hypertension' in the peri-operative setting is difficult. However, at the time of writing, upper limits range from 140/90 mmHg in the USA to 160/100 mmHg in the UK (see also Chapter 40, 'Hypertensive patient').

What are the causes of intra-operative hypertension?

> **Patient factors:**
  • Pre-existing uncontrolled hypertension:
    essential hypertension (90% of cases)
    secondary hypertension (e.g. Conn's syndrome, phaeochromocytoma, renal artery stenosis or pre-eclampsia in pregnant patients).
  • Disease states exacerbated by surgery (e.g. thyroid storm or the Cushing's reflex in the head-injured patient with raised intracranial pressures).
> **Anaesthetic factors:**
  • Inadequate depth of anaesthesia
  • Inadequate analgesia
  • Inadequate ventilation causing hypercapnia or hypoxia
  • Overdosing of vasopressor drugs causing iatrogenic hypertension
  • Malignant hyperpyrexia (rare)

How would you manage such a case?

> **Pre-operative:** An assessment should identify and optimise patient factors prior to elective surgery.
> **Intra-operative:** This requires an assessment to identify the cause followed by the required intervention, e.g. increase depth of anaesthesia, supplemental analgesia. Administration of antihypertensive medications may be required intra-operatively.
  Drugs that can be used to bring down BP in the acute setting include:
  • β-Blockers – esmolol is an ultra-short-acting agent given by infusion. Labetalol has α and β effects and is typically given as slow boluses titrated to effect.
  • Hydralazine – a directly acting vasodilator (arteries > veins) that can be administered if β-blockers are contraindicated.
  • GTN – a short-acting vasodilator (veins > arteries), and tolerance develops within 24 hours.
  • Sodium nitroprusside – an arteriolar vasodilator. It is light sensitive and prolonged use can lead to cyanide accumulation.
  • Remifentanil – a synthetic opioid that causes a decrease in mean arterial pressure and heart rate. Profound bradycardia can limit its use.

62. HYPOTENSION

It is hard to write a generic answer to this critical incident, as the answer you give in the exam will be tailored to the specific case presented to you. For example, it may be appropriate to discuss cardiac tamponade as a cause of hypotension in a trauma patient but it would not be appropriate as a common cause of hypotension in a 16-year-old undergoing an appendicectomy.

Approach this question using the physiological formula for calculation of mean arterial pressure (MAP):

MAP = Cardiac Output × Systemic Vascular Resistance (SVR)
MAP = (Heart Rate × Stroke Volume) × SVR

Thus, physiologically, hypotension may be secondary to reduced cardiac output, reduced SVR or a combination of both.

What are the causes of a low cardiac output?	> Bradycardia, e.g. β-blocker, opioids, vagal response, hypoxia > Arrhythmias, e.g. electrolyte imbalances, valvular or ischaemic heart disease > Reduced circulating volume or venous return (preload), e.g. hypovolaemia, cardiac tamponade, aorto-caval compression or tension pneumothorax > Impaired myocardial contractility, e.g. ischaemia, hypoxia, acidosis > Increased afterload, e.g. aortic stenosis (reduces left ventricular ejection fraction) or pulmonary embolism
What are the causes of a low SVR?	> Drugs, e.g. intravenous anaesthetic induction agents, vasodilators, α-receptor blockers > Spinal and epidural anaesthesia, via sympathetic blockade > Local mediators, e.g. potassium, nitric oxide > Hypercapnia > Pyrexia > Sepsis > Anaphylaxis
How would you manage intra-operative hypotension?	*Your management should be tailored to the likely causes. State that this is an anaesthetic emergency and that you would call for senior anaesthetic assistance.* > Administer 100% O_2 to maintain tissue oxygenation. > Recheck measurement and ensure invasive monitoring equipment is correctly positioned relative to patient. > Check what the surgeons are doing, e.g. exclude a sudden blood loss, surgical caval compression and ensure normal abdominal insufflation pressures.

> Correct the physiology by maintaining cardiac output and SVR which, depending on the cause of hypotension, may require any of the following interventions:
>   • Fluid challenge, e.g. 10mL/kg of crystalloid or colloid. Assess response and repeat as necessary. Transfuse blood if indicated.
>   • Vasoconstrictors, e.g. phenylephrine, metaraminol or noradrenaline.
>   • Inotropes, e.g. ephedrine, dobutamine, dopexamine, milrinone.
>   • Treat arrhythmias, e.g. electrolyte correction, anti-arrhythmics.

If hypotension becomes resistant to treatment, consider early use of cardiac output monitoring devices to guide further therapy. Remember that even short periods of intra-operative hypotension may have consequences on end-organ function.

Decide on appropriate post-operative care in the critical care unit if indicated.

63. HYPOXIA

This is an anaesthetic emergency that requires rapid detection and management in order to prevent patient harm. Examiners will expect a well-rehearsed drill and anything less will raise serious concerns. A structured approach is required.

What is hypoxia?

Definition: Arterial O_2 saturation < 90% or PaO_2 < 8 kP_a

> **Detection:**
>   • Pulse oximetry
>   • Cyanosis occurs at SaO_2 < 85% or PaO_2 < 6.7 kP_a
>   • Correlates with deoxygenated Hb > 5 g/dL

> **Associated:**
>   • Changes in BP or changes in HR
>   • Altered mental state
>   • Late signs: myocardial ischaemia, arrhythmias, bradycardia, hypotension and cardiac arrest

What are the causes of hypoxia?

> Low FiO_2 (hypoxic hypoxia)
>   • Relative (inadequate for patient's condition)
>   • Absolute (problems delivering O_2 to circuit)
> Inadequate alveolar minute ventilation
> $\dot{V}/\dot{Q}$ mismatch
> Anatomical shunt
> Anaemia (anaemic hypoxia)
> Low cardiac output (stagnant hypoxia)
> Histotoxic hypoxia (e.g. cyanide poisoning or carbon monoxide)
> Excess metabolic O_2 demand

Clinical causes:
> Inadequate alveolar minute ventilation
> Obstructed airway
> Endobronchial/oesophageal intubation
> Increased alveolar-arterial gradient
> Pre-existing lung disease (e.g. COPD and pulmonary fibrosis)
> Pneumothorax
> Pulmonary oedema
> Aspiration
> Atelectasis
> Pulmonary embolism
> Low cardiac output

Prevention:
> Check anaesthetic machine
> O_2 analyser and alarms
> Adequate ventilation (especially tidal volume)
> Maintain tidal volumes in normal range
> Monitor and adjust FiO_2
> Caution with spontaneous ventilation in lung disease

What are the causes of artificially low pulse oximeter saturation readings?

> Pulse oximeter malfunction – check waveform and probe position
> Hypothermia
> Poor peripheral circulation
> Artefacts – diathermy, motion, ambient lighting
> Dyes (e.g. methylene blue)

Describe your management of hypoxia.

State that this is an anaesthetic emergency and that you would call for senior anaesthetic assistance.

> Low SpO_2 on pulse oximetry is due to hypoxaemia until proved otherwise
> Increase FiO_2
> Verify FiO_2 increases – check oxygen analyser
> Verify pulse oximeter – check position, assess signal waveform and amplitude, and consider changing site
> Check other vital signs – heart rate, blood pressure, ECG, end-tidal CO_2
> Hand ventilate to assess lung compliance and confirm adequacy of ventilation
> Check chest movements and auscultate chest
> If an LMA is *in situ*, consider intubation to secure the airway
> Confirm endotracheal tube position and exclude endobronchial intubation
> Inform the surgeon, ask them to stop operating and to check retractors if applicable
> Check arterial blood gas to further define the degree of hypoxia

If saturations remain low, establish the cause and treat as appropriate:

> **Pulmonary:**
  • Pneumothorax
  • Bronchospasm
  • Lobar collapse
  • Mucous plugging
  • Aspiration
  • Massive atelectasis
  • Pulmonary embolism
  • Aspiration of foreign body
  • Acute pulmonary oedema
> **Extra-pulmonary:**
  • Low cardiac output
  • Anaemia
  • Intracardiac shunting (e.g. congenital heart disease)
  • Histotoxic hypoxia
> **Management options in persistent hypoxaemia:** Consider the use of the following interventions; the exact interventions will obviously depend upon the working clinical diagnosis.
  • Addition of PEEP
  • Ensure adequate tidal volume 6–10 mL/kg
  • Pulmonary toilet – suction endobronchial tube
  • Restore circulating blood volume
  • Bronchoscopy
  • Maintain cardiac output and Hb levels (Hb > 10 g/dL)
  • Transfer patient to supine position if applicable
  • Terminate surgery as soon as safely possible
  • Optimise ventilation and decide if extubation can be achieved safely or whether a period of prolonged ventilation will be required, this will depend on diagnosis
  • Arrange check CXR
  • Arrange transfer to ICU for further management
  • Document sequence of events in patient's medical records and complete critical incident form

64. INTRA-ARTERIAL INJECTION

Inadvertent intra-arterial injection is now a relatively rare occurrence, nevertheless it remains an anaesthetic emergency requiring prompt and effective management. The consequences of intra-arterial injection depend on the characteristics of the drug injected; sodium thiopentone, for example, precipitates into crystals, which cause intense vasospasm and may lead to arterial thrombosis.

What are the risk factors for intra-arterial injection?

> **Patient:**
> - Difficult intravenous access
> - Unconscious or anaesthetised patients
> - Positioning intravenous and intra-arterial access ports close to each other.

> **Site of cannulation:**
> - Antecubital fossa – unrecognised inadvertent cannulation of the brachial artery or aberrant ulnar artery
> - Dorsum of the hand – inadvertent cannulation of superficial branches of the radial artery.

How would you recognise inadvertent intra-arterial injection of thiopentone?

> Awake patients will complain of pain on injection, which should always be taken seriously. Intra-arterial injection may be associated with other signs such as skin blanching leading to cyanosis secondary to arterial spasm.

> Severe ischaemia from vasospasm and intra-arterial thrombosis may lead to digital necrosis.

How would you manage an inadvertent intra-arterial injection?

State that this is an anaesthetic emergency and that you would call for senior anaesthetic assistance.

> Stop injecting the drug.
> Aim to dilute the drug, dilate the artery, prevent thrombosis and provide analgesia.
> Leave the cannula *in situ*.
> Dilute the drug by flushing the cannula with 0.9% NaCl or heparinised saline.
> Vasodilate the artery by administering papaverine 40–80 mg if available.
> Administer 1000 IU heparin to minimise thrombosis risk.
> 10 mL of 1% lignocaine will provide some analgesia and has vasodilator properties.

> Sympathetic blockade of the upper limb will provide both analgesia and vasodilatation.
  • Sympathectomy may be achieved via stellate ganglion block, interscalene block or axillary block.
  • Guanethedine block is also an option if expertise is available, and has the advantage of long-lasting therapeutic effect.
> Anticoagulation should be continued for 10–14 days.
> Consult with a vascular surgeon if necessary.
> Inform the patient, complete a critical incident report form and document in the medical notes the sequence of events and management.

65. LARYNGOSPASM

What is laryngospasm?

Laryngospasm is the reflex adduction of the vocal cords and occurs most commonly during lighter planes of anaesthesia. Direct or indirect stimulation of the larynx may precipitate laryngospasm:

> Direct stimulation, e.g. blood, mucus, laryngoscope or endotracheal tube.
> Indirect stimulation via another site, e.g. pain, cervical or anal stimulation.

Laryngospasm may present as intra-operative stridor or sudden difficulty in ventilating the un-intubated patient.

Left unchecked laryngospasm may result in:

> Complete upper airway obstruction
> Desaturation and hypoxaemia
> Negative-pressure pulmonary oedema.

What are the risk factors for laryngospasm?

> Pre-existing upper respiratory tract infection ('irritable airway').
> Smoking.
> Children are more susceptible than adults especially if asthmatic, chest infection within last 6 weeks, exposed to passive smoking.
> Inadequate depth of anaesthesia for either airway manipulation or for surgical stimulus.
> Soiling of the vocal cords, e.g. blood.
> Upper airway surgery, e.g. tonsilectomy.

How would you manage a case of laryngospasm?

State that this is an anaesthetic emergency and that you would call for senior anaesthetic assistance.

> Remove the stimulus.
> Apply 100% O_2.
> Apply positive pressure to the airway to assist inspiration.
> If the above measures fail, deepen anaesthesia rapidly, e.g. administer a bolus of propofol at a dose appropriate to the patient.
> If deepening of anaesthesia fails, administer 1–2 mg/kg of suxamethonium to relax the vocal cords. If IV access is impossible, give 4 mg/kg i.m.
> Reintubation may be necessary. This will depend on the situation, patient and operation. Remember that laryngospasm may recur on re-extubation.
> Ensure documentation of the event and completion of a critical incident form.

66. LOCAL ANAESTHETIC TOXICITY

Over the last decade there have been significant improvements in the delivery of regional anaesthesia including ultrasound-guided nerve blockade, which allows accurate delivery of local anaesthetics and the introduction of less cardiotoxic local anaesthetics such as levobupivacaine and ropivacaine. Nevertheless, local anaesthetic (LA) toxicity remains an ever-present risk and as such, the emergency management is a core topic. The Association of Anaesthetists of Great Britain and Ireland (AAGBI) has produced guidelines for the management of severe local anaesthetic toxicity, and examiners will expect a clear and concise reproduction of these guidelines in an exam situation.

Factors to consider in the development of LA toxicity include the LA itself, site of injection, speed of absorption and the consequent rate of rise in plasma concentration. The physiological and metabolical state of the patient may also play a role, e.g. hypoxia, hypercarbia and acidosis all potentiate cardiotoxicity.

For all these reasons, the actual maximum recommended dose of LA needs to be interpreted in the correct clinical context. However, examiners would expect you to know the recommended maximum doses:

Overview

LA	Max dose	With added vasoconstrictor
Lignocaine	3 mg/kg	7 mg/kg (adrenaline)
Bupivacaine	2 mg/kg	–
Levobupivacaine	2 mg/kg	–
Ropivacaine	3 mg/kg	–
Cocaine	3 mg/kg	–
Amethocaine	1.5 mg/kg	–
Prilocaine	6 mg/kg	8 mg/kg (felypressin)

What are the clinical features of LA toxicity?

Clinical features depend on plasma concentration of LA. For example, early symptoms in an awake patient with a plasma lignocaine concentration of 2–4 µg/mL may include light-headedness, tinnitus, circumoral tingling and tongue numbness. Plasma levels between 5 and 10 µg/mL will lead to visual disturbances, agitation and muscular twitching. Plasma levels above 10 µg/mL may lead to tonic–clonic convulsions followed by coma and respiratory arrest. At plasma levels of 15 and 25 µg/mL cardiotoxicity will result, leading to cardiovascular collapse and development of malignant arrhythmias (conduction blocks, ventricular tachyarrhythmias and asystole).

Describe your management of LA toxicity.	*State that this is an anaesthetic emergency and that you would call for senior anaesthetic assistance and make a rapid but thorough assessment of the patient.*

> Stop injecting the LA.
> Maintain and, if necessary, secure the airway with a cuffed endotracheal tube.
> Administer 100% oxygen and ensure adequate lung ventilation (hyperventilation may be of benefit by increasing pH).
> Confirm or establish IV access.
> Control seizures using a benzodiazepine (e.g. lorazepam) or use small incremental doses of thiopentone or propofol.
> Assess cardiovascular status throughout. Arterial line insertion would be of benefit.

Management of cardiac arrest

> Commence cardiopulmonary resuscitation (CPR) following Advanced Life Support (ALS) protocols.
> Manage arrhythmias using the same ALS protocols, recognising that arrhythmias may be refractory to treatment and prolonged resuscitation (several hours) may be necessary.
> It may be appropriate to consider other treatment options:
> • Consider cardiopulmonary bypass if available.
> • Consider treatment with lipid emulsion.

Treatment of cardiac arrest with lipid emulsion

Approximate doses for a 70 kg patient are given in italics:

> Administer an intravenous bolus of Intralipid® 20% (1.5 mL/kg) over 1 min (*100 mL bolus*).
> Continue CPR.
> Start an infusion of Intralipid® 20% at 0.25 mL/kg/min (*400 mL over 20 min*).
> Repeat the bolus injection (*100 mL*) of Intralipid® 20% twice at 5 min intervals if an adequate circulation has not been restored.
> After another 5 min, increase the rate of infusion to 0.5 mL/kg/min if an adequate circulation has not been restored (*400 mL over 10 min*).
> Continue infusion until a stable and adequate circulation has been restored.

Remember

> Continue CPR throughout treatment with lipid emulsion.
> Recovery from LA-induced cardiac arrest may take >1 hour.
> Propofol is not a suitable substitute for Intralipid® 20%.
> Replace your supply of Intralipid® 20% after use.

Follow-up action

> Inform the patient of the event, answer any questions and ensure medical documentation is complete.
> Complete a local hospital critical incident form.
> Report case to the National Patient Safety Agency (NPSA) (via www.npsa.nhs.uk).

67. MALIGNANT HYPERPYREXIA

It is safe to say that the majority of us are unlikely to ever experience a case of malignant hyperpyrexia (MH) during our careers. However, malignant hyperpyrexia remains a life-threatening anaesthetic emergency with a mortality rate of approximately 10%.

Describe the pathophysiology of MH.

> Malignant hyperpyrexia (or malignant hyperthermia) is an autosomal dominant disorder of skeletal muscle. Its genetics are complex, with over 15 causative mutations; chromosome 19 is most commonly involved. The incidence of genetic susceptibility is now thought to be between 1:5000 and 1:10000.
> The various gene mutations affect the calcium release channels in the sarcoplasmic reticulum (SR). The ryanodine receptor (a calcium release channel) fails and intracellular calcium levels increase up to 500-fold, leading to sustained muscle contraction.
> MH is an anaesthetic-related disorder. All inhalational agents and depolarising muscle relaxants can trigger the abnormal handling of calcium within skeletal muscles.

How would you recognise MH?

The successful management of MH begins with its prompt recognition. MH presents in two main ways, either with excessive muscle rigidity or with signs of hypermetabolism.

> **Excessive muscle rigidity:** This often presents at induction as masseter spasm following suxamethonium, although generalised muscle rigidity may also occur. With ongoing muscle rigidity rhabdomyolysis occurs, serum potassium (K^+) increases (potentially causing arrhythmias), creatinine kinase (CK) increases and acute renal failure can ensue.
> **Hypermetabolism:** This occurs due to the increased ATP demand required to fuel the abnormal contractions and membrane calcium pumps. The earliest signs include:

  • Unexplained tachycardia
  • Tachypnoea (in a spontaneously breathing patient)
  • Rising end-tidal CO_2 ($ETCO_2$)
  • Falling arterial O_2 tensions (PaO_2).

With time, the patient's temperature rises, sometimes by as much as 1 °C every 10 minutes. As more oxygen is consumed, hypoxaemia and cyanosis occur, giving rise to a metabolic acidosis. As CO_2 levels continue to rise, a respiratory acidosis develops.

Describe your management of MH.

State that this is an anaesthetic emergency.

> Call for senior help urgently and inform the theatre team that you have an emergency. Also, call for help from any free operating department practitioners (ODPs).

> Disconnect patient from the anaesthetic machine immediately and begin hand hyperventilation with 100% oxygen (to reduce $PaCO_2$). Use O_2 drawn from an alternative source to the anaesthetic machine so that it is free of inhalational agents. With a new circuit, use high flows to wash out the inhalational agents and CO_2.

> Maintain anaesthesia using intravenous agents (e.g. propofol).

> Ask an ODP to bring and prepare the 'vapour-free' anaesthetic machine for use (every department should have one and you must know where it is kept). Ventilate with this when ready.

> Send assistants to prepare dantrolene sodium urgently. Each vial contains 20 mg dantrolene and 3 g mannitol and this crystalline mixture must be mixed with 60 mL water. When it is ready, give 1 mg/kg IV. Repeat dose every 5–10 min until the tachycardia, hypercapnia and temperature start to subside. On average 3 mg/kg is needed but up to 10 mg/kg may be required. Doses may need to be repeated in the subsequent 48 hours if the reaction recurs, although this is rare. Dantrolene works within skeletal muscles by preventing the release of calcium from the sarcoplasmic reticulum.

> Ask the surgeons to conclude surgery as fast as possible.

> Instigate active cooling measures. The surgeons are well placed to do this. Use cold intravenous fluids, cold body cavity lavages, ice packs to groin and axillae, and cooling blankets.

> Appoint someone to record observations, drug doses, times, etc.

> Gain sufficient intravenous access, site an arterial cannula, temperature probe and urinary catheter.

> Manage hyperkalaemia and acidosis expectantly, guided by regular arterial blood gas analysis and electrolyte measurements. Use insulin/dextrose and bicarbonate infusions as appropriate.

> Send regular clotting profiles to check for disseminated intravascular coagulopathy (DIC) and treat appropriately (e.g. with fresh frozen plasma).

> Manage rhabdomyolysis expectantly guided by renal function, CK levels and urinary myoglobin concentrations. Maintain urine output at 2 mL/kg/h with fluid and diuretics to limit renal tubular damage.

> Finally, when stable, transfer patient to ITU.

> **H**elp
> **O**xygen
> **S**top inhalational agents/**S**top surgery
> **P**ropofol infusion
> **I**ntravenous dantrolene
> **T**emperature regulation
> **A**ddress metabolic derangement
> **L**iaise with ITU

Describe your subsequent management.

> Counsel the patient and their relatives about events and the implications of a potential diagnosis of MH.

> Document events in clinical notes and inform the GP.

> Suggest a MedicAlert bracelet.

> Patients must be referred to St James's University Hospital MH investigation unit in Leeds, where a muscle biopsy will be taken for '*in vitro* muscle contracture testing' (muscle tissue is exposed to caffeine and halothane, which reduce the threshold for muscle contraction). This is the gold standard diagnostic test for MH.

68. NEEDLESTICK INJURY

Needlestick injury can have huge implications for the individual involved, not only in terms of disease transmission and the effect it may have on employment but also because of the anxiety and psychological strain it can cause while waiting for test results. This question requires you to demonstrate knowledge of associated risk factors and methods used to minimise them. It may explore your management of the event, which should focus on ensuring your safety and that of your patient, using local guidelines.

You are suturing a central venous line in a 36-year-old male diagnosed with pancreatitis when you inadvertently sustain a needlestick injury. What immediate action would you take?

> Call for help so that someone can relieve you and look after the patient.
> Encourage free bleeding of the wound.
> Immediately wash the wound with soap and water (do not scrub or suck).
> Follow local policy and inform occupational health to report the incident and to seek further advice (out of hours go to your A&E department).
> Establish whether you should start to take post-exposure prophylaxis (PEP) to HIV by performing a risk assessment of the patient.

How would you perform a 'risk assessment' of your patient?

A risk assessment aims to identify those individuals who are more likely to be infected with HIV, hepatitis B (HBV) or hepatitis C (HCV). Transmission rates are 0.3% for HIV, 3% for HCV and 30% HBV.

Explain to the patient what has happened and that for your safety, a formal risk assessment is very important.

Ensure that this is done in private to maintain confidentiality.

If the patient lacks capacity to give consent to testing, e.g. is sedated on ICU, then current GMC guidance counsels against testing until consent can be gained. This is a contentious area and local policy should be followed.

> **History:**
> • HIV, HBV and HCV status
> • Sexuality: homosexual intercourse or casual partners including prostitutes
> • Use of intravenous drugs and needle sharing
> • Tattoos
> • Blood transfusions abroad or multiple blood transfusions
> • History of jaundice
> • Recent holiday or residency in a country with a high HIV incidence.
> **Examination:**
> • Tattoos
> • Needle track marks
> • Lymphadenopathy.
> **Investigations:** Gain the patient's consent to take blood for HIV, HBV and HCV testing (the patient must be given appropriate counselling prior to this – follow your local hospital protocol on 'donor' counselling).

What further steps would you undertake?

> Have your blood taken shortly after the injury to confirm your current status (follow-up blood tests will be required later).
> Commence PEP if patient deemed to be high risk. Ideally, this should be started within 1 hour of injury, and should consist of a triple-therapy regime of zidovudine, lamivudine and indinavir that is taken for 4 weeks. Unfortunately, these agents can cause serious side effects such as jaundice, diabetes, vomiting and profound fatigue.
> Establish your hepatitis B status. All healthcare professionals should be vaccinated prior to starting work. If you are a known responder, you should be given a hepatitis B vaccine booster. If you are susceptible, you should be given an accelerated hepatitis B vaccination course along with hepatitis B immunoglobulin. There is currently no official treatment for suspected or confirmed exposure to hepatitis C.
> Inform your clinical lead, as a suspected exposure to HIV, HBV or HCV may preclude you from performing certain exposure-prone procedures. The Department of Health has stated airway manipulation using gloves is not an exposure-prone procedure.
> Seek counselling.
> Complete a critical incident form.

What are the major risk factors associated with the transmission of blood-borne viruses?

> **Exposure to high-risk fluids:**
  • High-risk fluids: blood, amniotic, peritoneal, pleural, pericardial and cerebrospinal fluid, semen and vaginal secretions
  • Low-risk fluids: faeces, urine, saliva and vomit
> **Mechanism of injury**
  • Percutaneous injury (e.g. with needles)
  • Exposure of broken skin (e.g. cuts)
  • Exposure of mucous membrane (e.g. splash on the eye).
> **Type of instrument:** Hollow bore needles carry higher risk than solid needles.
> **Patient:** Blood or fluid from terminally ill patients or those with a high viral load is more contagious.

What precautions can be taken to reduce risk of infection?

> Universal precautions when performing any exposure-prone procedures: gloves, mask and goggles.
> Avoid resheathing needles and use sharps bin to dispose of equipment promptly.
> Cover open skin lesions (but ideally avoid patient contact).
> Avoid mouth-to-mouth ventilation.
> Use of HMEF filters on breathing circuits between patients.
> Hepatitis B vaccination of healthcare professionals.
> Exposure protection plan and management plan.

69. POST-DURAL PUNCTURE HEADACHE

Describe the common causes and presentation of a post-dural puncture headache (PDPH).

Dural puncture is intentional in subarachnoid anaesthesia and a recognised complication of epidural placement. Puncturing the dura can result in leakage of CSF from the tear, a fall in ICP and sagging of the brain in the skull vault, which can lead to the development of a debilitating postural headache. The headache usually occurs within 72 hours of dural puncture, is classically severe, frontal/occipital/retrobulbar and may radiate into the neck and shoulders. The pain is worse on sitting or standing and improved by lying down. There may be associated nausea and vomiting, photophobia, tinnitus, hearing loss, vertigo, paraesthesia of the scalp or upper and lower limbs. In every instance, other causes of headache must be considered and excluded.

What is the incidence of PDPH?

The incidence of accidental dural puncture during epidural anaesthesia is 0–2.6% and is inversely proportional to the experience of the anaesthetist. Incidence of post-dural puncture headache (PDPH) following spinal depends on the type and gauge of needle used: with 25 g Whitacre incidence is 0–14.5%, 24 g Sprotte 0–9.6%.

The most common place you will encounter dural punctures and PDPH is in the maternity unit because of the large numbers of epidurals sited in labouring women.

You are inserting an epidural into a woman in early labour. You suspect you may have accidentally punctured the dura. Describe your management.

Management of an accidental dural puncture can be classified as immediate, early and late:

Immediate management:
> Confirm dural puncture: this may be extremely obvious if there is CSF leaking briskly from the Tuohy needle! Otherwise CSF can be identified by feeling the temperature of the fluid on your un-gloved hand or dip the fluid with a urine dipstix:
  • CSF warm, pH 7.5–8.5, trace/+ glucose, +/++ protein
  • Saline cool, pH 5–7.5, no glucose, no protein.
> Once dural puncture is confirmed, there are two management options available:
  • Remove the needle/catheter and re-site the epidural at a different interspace. Run the epidural as needed following this, but beware of intrathecal spread of local anaesthetic. Only an anaesthetist should give top ups.

- Continue and thread the epidural catheter into the subarachnoid space. This is the authors' favoured approach because analgesia will be excellent, there is no risk of repeating the dural puncture on further attempts, there is some small evidence that fibroblast proliferation around the catheter reduces the chance of PDPH and the risk of unpredictable subarachnoid spread of a re-sited epidural is eliminated. The disadvantages of this option are that further management of the spinal catheter is labour intensive for the anaesthetist: the patient may not have an infusion/PCEA; instead all top up doses must be administered by an anaesthetist to avoid a high spinal.
  - o When topping up the spinal catheter, be cautious, starting with doses of 1–2 mL of standard low-dose mixture (0.125% bupivacaine + 2 µg/mL fentanyl) to 'get a feel' for how much each woman will need. Titrate dose to block height and effect.
  - o Clearly label the catheter as a 'SPINAL CATHETER'. Inform a senior anaesthetist, the midwife and the woman of events, and document events in her notes.
  - o If the woman does not develop a headache during labour, she can labour as normal. If she does, assisted delivery may be advised to avoid excessive pushing that might worsen the CSF leak.
  - o If the woman proceeds to theatre, the spinal catheter can be used to 'top up' for a caesarean or assisted delivery, but this should be done with due caution as the spread of bupivacaine may be different via an epidural catheter than through a spinal needle.

There is a 70% chance that the parturient who suffers accidental dural puncture will go on to develop a PDPH.

Early Management:

Arrange daily follow-up for the woman by an anaesthetist and give her written information, e.g. OAA leaflet.

Late management of PDPH:

Conservative treatment
> Bed rest. Most PDPHs resume spontaneously after around 10 days. Traditional teaching encouraged fluid administration, but this has not been shown to be of benefit, although it is advisable to avoid dehydration.
> Avoid raising ICP: prescribe laxatives to all with PDPH to avoid the need to strain at stool. Advise patients to avoid lifting heavy loads or other activities that will cause straining.

Analgesia
> The woman should be given regular simple analgesia and opioids if needed (NB: do not give codeine to breastfeeding women).
> Caffeine, sumatriptan, abdominal binders: none of these traditional treatments has been shown to be effective.

Epidural blood patch
> If the woman develops a PDPH, consider offering a blood patch to treat it. Blood patches should be performed ≥24 hours after the initial injury, before this time they are thought to be less effective.
> The most senior anaesthetist available should perform the blood patch.
> Do not perform if the woman is pyrexial or showing signs of infection.
> Ask the woman to feed the baby and pass urine prior to coming for the blood patch.

> Perform the blood patch as close to the puncture site as possible, ideally one space below.
> Aim to inject 20–30 mL blood slowly. Pain may result due to arachnoid irritation. Flush the needle with 2 mL saline before removing it. Women often complain of back pain and should be warned of this beforehand.
> Keep woman lying flat for 2 hours and then allow her to mobilise cautiously.
> A single blood patch effects a permanent cure in around 50% of patients. Around 40% require a second procedure. By the natural history of a dural puncture, the headache will resolve in most patients by 10 days, even without treatment.

Offer the woman a follow-up after discharge to ensure there are no ongoing complications.

70. ST SEGMENT CHANGES

What is the significance of ST segment change?

The ST segment of the ECG represents repolarisation of the ventricles. Changes in the appearance of the ST segments are caused by myocardial ischaemia or myocardial infarction. In the face of ischaemia, ST segment depression or elevation may occur relative to the isoelectric line. Movement away from the isoelectric line of ≥1 mm is significant.

Intra-operative ST segment changes require rapid detection and management in order to correct and optimise coronary blood flow and reduce myocardial work. Intra-operatively, the most common causes of myocardial ischaemia are rate-related ischaemia and hypotension.

How would you manage an anaesthetised patient with ST segment changes?

> **Immediate management:**
  - Give 100% oxygen.
  - Call for help and inform the surgeons of the need to conclude surgery as soon as possible.
  - Perform a rapid but thorough assessment of the patient, looking for precipitating causes, e.g. hypoxia, tachycardia, hypotension and acute blood loss. Address any correctable problems.
  - Ensure adequate coronary perfusion pressure (increase aortic diastolic pressure), optimise arterial oxygen content (increase FiO_2 and ensure normal Hb concentration), optimise coronary blood flow (increase diastolic time and promote coronary vasodilatation) and reduce myocardial oxygen consumption (reduce heart rate and force of contraction). Vasoactive drugs such as intravenous nitrates, β-blockers or vasopressors may be required.

> **Early management:**
  - Consider additional monitoring: arterial line, cardiac output monitoring and central line if there seems to be physiological deterioration as a result of cardiac ischaemia.
  - If relevant, use cardiac output monitoring to guide fluid and inotropic therapy.
  - Check electrolytes and Hb, correct any abnormalities.

> **Post-operatively:**
  - Following the operation, transfer the patient to an area of high dependency care for observation and investigation.
  - Perform a 12-lead ECG and if abnormal, continue to take serial ECGs.
  - Repeat U&Es and FBC and glucose.
  - Take blood for a troponin I level at 6 and 12 hours after the event.
  - Request an urgent review by the on call cardiologist/medics. Do not wait for the results of blood tests before referral. Full anticoagulation/thrombolysis is unlikely to be possible immediately post-operatively and the patient may need urgent angiography.
  - Document events clearly in the notes.

71. TACHYARRHYTHMIAS

What are the causes of intra-operative tachyarrythmias?

> **Patient factors:** All patients undergoing anaesthesia and surgery are at risk of intra-operative arrhythmias. However, certain patients are at increased risk:
> • Pre-existing cardiac disease, e.g. ischaemic heart disease or valvular heart disease
> • Pre-existing arrhythmia, e.g. atrial fibrillation or Wolff–Parkinson–White syndrome
> • Pre-existing electrolyte disturbances, e.g. diuretic-induced hypokalaemia and hypomagnesaemia
> • Endocrine disease, e.g. thyrotoxicosis.

> **Anaesthetic factors:** General and regional anaesthetic techniques can have significant effects on cardiac function:
> • Drug-induced alteration in cardiac preload, contractility and afterload
> • Effects on coronary perfusion pressure
> • Effects on myocardial irritability
> • Effects on autonomic nervous system
> • Effects of hypoxia and hypercapnia
> • Electrolyte disturbances (either pre-existing or iatrogenic from fluid therapy)
> • Effects of intravascular devices (e.g. central venous lines) advanced too far and entering the right atrium

> **Surgical factors:**
> • Effects of pneumoperitoneum related to laparoscopic surgery, e.g. vagal response, reduced venous return, fall in cardiac index or rise in SVR
> • Effects of hypercapnia related to laparoscopic surgery, e.g. arrhythmias
> • Effects of rapid fluid shifts
> • Systemic inflammatory response syndrome (SIRS) induced by tissue trauma

The combination of patient, anaesthetic and surgical factors may lead to the development of intra-operative arrhythmias. The arrhythmias may be benign (e.g. occasional ventricular ectopics) or potentially malignant arrhythmias may develop (e.g. ventricular tachycardia).

Describe your management of an intra-operative tachyarrhythmia.

Management of intra-operative tachyarrhythmia follows general principles applicable to all tachyarrhythmias and specific treatments for certain types of tachyarrhythmias.

General management principles:
> Consider calling for assistance depending on the haemodynamic consequences of the arrhythmia.
> Diagnose the arrhythmia and establish the haemodynamic consequences – check blood pressure and end-tidal CO_2.

> Attempt to identify and treat the cause of the arrhythmia, e.g. adjust CVP line tip position or correct electrolyte disturbances.
> Attempt to maximise myocardial oxygen delivery by maintaining arterial oxygen content and coronary perfusion pressure.
> Check and correct electrolyte disturbances (potassium and magnesium): arterial blood gas analysis is the fastest method of obtaining potassium concentration (if hypokalaemia is present, in the majority of cases hypomagnesaemia will also be present).
> Attempt to correct any identified acid–base abnormalities detected on arterial blood gas.

Specific management:
> **Broad complex tachycardia (VF/VT/SVT with aberrant conduction)**
  • If there is no pulse, follow ALS protocol.
  • If there is a pulse assess the haemodynamic consequences:
  • **Systolic <90 mmHg/heart rate >150:** Synchronised DC cardioversion (up to three shocks). If refractory consider amiodarone 150 mg over 10 minutes followed by 300 mg over 1 hour and repeat shock if necessary. Consider lignocaine and overdrive pacing.
  • **Systolic >90 mmHg/heart rate <150:** Correct K^+ (>4.0 mmol/L) and Mg^{2+} (>1.0 mmol/L). Administer amiodarone 150 mg IV over 10 minutes or lignocaine 50 mg over 2 minutes repeated every 5 minutes up to a total dose of 200 mg.
> **Narrow complex tachycardia (SVT/atrial flutter)**
  • If there is no pulse, follow the ALS protocol.
  • If the rhythm is atrial fibrillation (AF), follow AF algorithm.
  • If there is a pulse and atrial fibrillation is excluded, assess the haemodynamic consequences:
  • **Systolic <90 mmHg/ventricular rate >200:** Synchronised DC cardioversion (up to three shocks). Consider amiodarone 150 mg over 10 minutes followed by 300 mg over 1 hour and repeat shock if necessary.
  • **Systolic >90 mmHg/ventricular rate <200:** Attempt vagal manoeuvre (e.g. carotid sinus massage). Consider adenosine boluses 6 mg, followed by up to three 12 mg doses. If resistant, consider use of esmolol, amiodarone, digoxin or verapamil.
> **Atrial fibrillation**
  Management depends on the time of onset (i.e. acute/chronic AF and subsequent risk of systemic embolisation if sinus rhythm is restored), ventricular rate and the haemodynamic consequences:

Critical AF, ventricular rate >150, hypotension and impaired perfusion
> Heparise if feasible (note risk of intra-operative bleeding)
> Administer synchronised DC cardioversion
> Administer amiodarone 300 mg IV over 1 hour followed by 900 mg over the following 23 hours

Intermediate AF, ventricular rate 100–150
If associated with haemodynamic compromise:

> Onset <24 hours: Heparinise and administer synchronised DC cardioversion. Consider amiodarone IV 300 mg over 1 hour.
> Onset >24 hours: Control rate initially with amiodarone IV 300 mg over 1 hour. Heparinise and later perform synchronised DC cardioversion.

If associated with normal haemodynamics:

> Onset <24 hours: Heparinise and administer amiodarone IV 300 mg over 1 hour. Consider flecainide. Synchronised DC cardioversion may be required.

> Onset >24 hours: Control rate initially with digoxin, verapamil or β-blockers. Heparinise and later perform synchronised DC cardioversion.

Low-risk AF, ventricular Rate <100 with good perfusion

> Onset <24 hours: Heparinise and administer amiodarone IV 300 mg over 1 hour. Consider flecainide.

> Onset >24 hours: Heparinise and then later perform synchronised DC cardioversion.

Post-operative:

All patients who have suffered significant intra-operative arrhythmias should have cardiac monitoring in the initial post-operative period (including 12-lead ECG) and relevant cardiac follow-up if indicated.

ALS protocols have not been covered here but are likely to be examined in the OSCE.

72. VENOUS AIR EMBOLISM (VAE)

Venous air embolism (VAE) is a potential complication of many surgical procedures. The clinical features range from sub-clinical to life-threatening cardiovascular collapse depending upon the rate and volume of gas that is entrained into the circulation.

Examiners will expect an understanding of the types of procedures that are associated with an increased risk of VAE, and also the ability to diagnose and manage the problem.

What procedures are associated with a high risk of VAE?

> Neurosurgery, particularly surgery in the sitting position and surgery involving the cranium and dura.
> Laparoscopic surgery with risk of direct intravascular gas insufflation.
> Head and neck surgery with large areas of tissue exposed, often with vessels at subatmospheric pressure.
> Orthopaedic surgery, e.g. polytrauma, cementing and reaming in long bone surgery
> Insertion of intravascular devices, e.g. central venous cannulation.

How can you diagnose VAE?

Symptoms and signs are primarily those of cardiovascular collapse (hypotension, tachycardia, arrhythmias and arterial desaturation) caused by the air embolus acting as an intracardiac air lock. In the correct clinical setting, suspicion for VAE must always remain high. In certain high-risk procedures (e.g. neurosurgery in the sitting position) monitoring should be used electively to aid early VAE detection and may include the following:

> Listen for audible hissing as gas enters the circulation.
> ECG: VAE is associated with an increase in pulmonary vascular resistance and the development of right ventricular dysfunction causing arrhythmias and possibly a right ventricular strain pattern.
> Capnography: fall in end-tidal CO_2.
> CVP increases.
> Precordial stethoscope: classic 'millwheel murmur'. This is insensitive and a late sign.
> Pulmonary artery pressure increases.
> Oesophageal Doppler is extremely useful in early detection of VAE.
> Transoesophageal echocardiography (TOE): Possibly the gold standard. Allows localisation of air to a specific cardiac chamber while enabling assessment of cardiac function.

What is the management of a suspected VAE?

State that this is an anaesthetic emergency, and that you would call for senior anaesthetic assistance and make a rapid but thorough assessment of the patient.

> Inform the surgeon who may be able to prevent further embolisation by compression of the surgical site or flooding the surgical site with saline.
> Administer 100% oxygen and discontinue nitrous oxide, which will increase bubble size due to its high solubility.
> Increase CVP by tilting the patient slightly head-down, administer fluid and increase PEEP.
> Position patient in left lateral head-down position if feasible, this may prevent embolisation into the pulmonary artery. In this position consider attempting to aspirate the air via a CVP line.
> Cardiovascular support with fluid and inotropic support may be required. CPR may also become necessary if the situation deteriorates.
> Terminate surgery as soon as safely possible.
> Arrange appropriate post-operative care (ITU or HDU).
> Document events and complete a critical incident form.
> Explain the event to the patient when possible.

INDEX